BASIC EXPERIMENTATION IN PSYCHOACOUSTICS

BASIC EXPERIMENTATION IN PSYCHOACOUSTICS

Alan M. Richards, Ph.D.
Associate Professor
Department of Speech and Theatre
Speech and Hearing Center
Herbert H. Lehman College
Bronx, New York

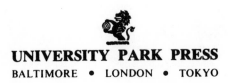

UNIVERSITY PARK PRESS
BALTIMORE • LONDON • TOKYO

UNIVERSITY PARK PRESS
International Publishers in Science and Medicine
Chamber of Commerce Building
Baltimore, Maryland 21202

Copyright © 1976 by University Park Press

Typeset by The Composing Room of Michigan, Inc.
Manufactured in the United States of America by
Universal Lithographers, Inc., and The Maple Press Co.

Library of Congress Cataloging in Publication Data

Richards, Alan M
    Basic experimentation in psychoacoustics.

    Bibliography: p.
    Includes index.
    1. Psychoacoustics. 2. Audiometry. I. Title.
QP461.R5   612'.85   76-7454
ISBN 0-8391-0884-2

contents

preface

This book is written primarily for students of audiology, practicing audiologists, and for persons outside the field of audiology who are concerned with hearing research. Psychoacoustics, besides playing an integral role in experimental and sensory psychology, provides the methodological and experimental foundations upon which many of the commonly used audiometric procedures are based. This dependence is seen from the simplest of audiometric tasks, that of determining an absolute threshold in quiet, to more complex tasks used in the diagnosis of site of auditory pathology. In the rapidly expanding field of audiology, where new information is being disseminated at an ever increasing rate, it is often the case that a full appreciation of the normal psychoacoustic phenomenon underlying the test development is not attained. The student or practitioner may become familiar with the clinical test, and may be able to interpret it. However, he or she may not fully appreciate the underlying principles or methodology. This book provides the student of audiology with a basic understanding of various psychoacoustic phenomena and the instrumentation and methods necessary to study these phenomena.

The book is designed to provide an integrated approach to the study of psychoacoustic experimentation. That is, each chapter is written to provide the introductory material in order to fully appreciate the next chapter. The book is divided into four chapters. Chapter 1 acquaints the student with basic terminology used in the field. Two sections are included. The first section defines terms dealing with stimulus parameters, test environment, and experimental methodology. The second section gives the definitions of basic psychoacoustic terms. Chapter 2 introduces basic equipment for psychoacoustic experimentation. Chapter 3 deals with how the various instruments in Chapter 2 may be interconnected in a logical sequence to produce a workable array of experimental apparatus. The primary objective of Chapter 4 is to demonstrate how to set up and conduct a psychoacoustic experiment. The format of the chapter is to first present introductory material for each of several classical psychoacoustic subject areas. This is followed by the presentation of several of the methods used to investigate the area. A detailed description of an illustrative experiment in the area is then offered. The primary intent of these experiments is to provide the student with a model that he or she may use in performing similar experiments. Each experiment includes step-by-step descriptions of the experimental apparatus arrangement, calibration procedures, methodological procedures and considerations, and data analysis information.

Acknowledgment is hereby made to several persons who were influential in the course of the development and editing of this book. My colleague, Dr. Allan C. Goodman, was very helpful in editing the manuscript. His aid and ideas are much appreciated. Chapter 2 was read for content by Robert Guinta of R. R. Guinta Associates. He has been extremely helpful to me in innumerable ways over the years. Mr. Jan Dunn photographed several of the pieces of apparatus. His help is most appreciated. My wife Ellen has, as always, served as editor, advisor, and inspiration. Her faith in my abilities has inspired me throughout the course of my career. I am deeply indebted to her.

To Brian

chapter 1

INTRODUCTION TO COMMONLY USED TERMS IN PSYCHOACOUSTICS

The student of psychoacoustics must be acquainted with introductory concepts and basic terminology. Without a working knowledge of these terms the task of designing an experiment in the field would be nearly impossible. Thus, this first chapter introduces the reader to basic terminology used in the design and execution of psychoacoustic experiments. The chapter is divided into two sections. The first deals with stimulus parameters, the test environment, and experimental methodology. The second deals with definitions of basic psychoacoustic phenomena.

1.1. TERMINOLOGY DEALING WITH STIMULUS PARAMETERS, THE TEST ENVIRONMENT, AND EXPERIMENTAL METHODOLOGY

Ambient noise: Ambient noise is the background noise in the test environment. In most experiments dealing with audition, the ambient noise should be kept to a minimum. Ambient noise may also be present in the instrumentation in the form of hum or hiss.

Amplification: Amplification is the process by which a signal of comparatively weak strength is applied to the input of an amplifier and appears at the output in increased strength. Although the signal at the output is greater than at the input, the waveforms should not differ. Amplification may be expressed as a direct ratio between the input and the output levels, but is more commonly described as a logarithmic ratio in terms of decibels (dB) gain. For example, if the input to an amplifier is

1

0.01 volt and the output is 10 volts, the input to output ratio is 1,000:1, which corresponds to a voltage gain of 60 dB.

Amplitude: The amplitude of a sound wave is related to the distance that the sound-producing body (vibrator) moves during vibration. The greater the distance from the null point, the greater the amplitude. *Instantaneous amplitude* refers to the excursion distance at any instant in time, while *peak amplitude* refers to the greatest displacement achieved by the sound source. The *RMS* (root-mean square) *amplitude* is a statistical average of all amplitudes at all times.

Anechoic chamber: An anechoic chamber is a specially designed room which is free of echoes because of its ability to absorb incident sound. Anechoic chambers are constructed so that the floor, walls, and ceiling are covered with wedges (usually fiberglass) which protrude into the room. A wire mesh platform suspended above the floor accomodates the test equipment and subjects. Figure 1.1 shows a photograph of such a chamber. An important use of these chambers in psychoacoustics is in sound localization studies. The room provides a facility where the subject may localize without the confounding effects of reverberation.

Artificial ear: See Coupler.

Attenuate: To attenuate is to make a signal less intense. In acoustics the attenuation process may be natural, as when sound is absorbed by room structures or when it passes through a boundary such as a wall. Sound is also naturally attenuated by increasing the distance from the sound source (−6 dB/doubling of distance). Sound may artificially be attenuated by devices called attenuators. Typically, in psychoacoustic experimentation, these devices are placed just before output transducers (earphones and loudspeakers) so that the voltage to the transducer may be reduced in decibel steps. The sound level output of the transducer is then reduced by an equivalent decibel amount. To increase attenuation is to decrease intensity. To decrease attenuation is to increase intensity.

Attenuation rate: In many instances the attenuation of an acoustic signal is not accomplished with a manual attenuator, but is under the control of a mechanical device called a recording attenuator. A recording attenuator is a motor-driven attenuator with a mechanical linkage between the attenuator and a pen recorder. Thus, the attenuation value at any instant in time may be graphically displayed. The rate of attenuation is constant and may be expressed in dB/second. The use of recording attenuators is quite common in psychacoustic research and in clinical audiology. There are generally used for threshold determination.

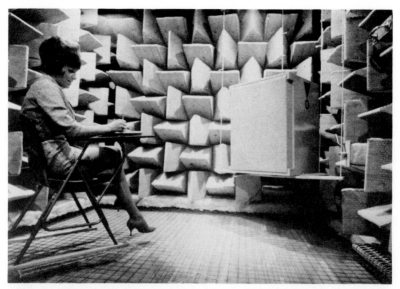

Figure 1.1. Photograph of the interior of an anechoic chamber. Courtesy of Industrial Acoustics Company, Inc.

Bandwidth: The bandwidth of a device is the range of frequencies within which the device remains above a specified level. Typically, the bandwidth in Hertz (Hz) extends from the points where the performance of the device is 3 dB below the average passband level. The bandwidth of a band of noise may also be specified by its 3 dB down (half-power) points. See Narrow-band noise and Frequency response.

Broad-band noise: Broad-band noise has a wide bandwidth which may extend over the entire audible spectrum. The most frequently used type of broad-band noise is referred to as "white-noise." White-noise consists of a continuous spectrum of frequencies with equal energy per cycle. In practice, the bandwidth of white-noise may be limited to between 6,000–7,000 Hz because of the limited frequency response of earphones.

Calibration: Calibration is the single most important factor in obtaining accurate, reliable, and meaningful data in an experiment or in the clinic. In general, calibration refers to the process by which the physical output characteristics of the apparatus are indicated as the various control dials are manipulated. For example, if an experiment is designed to determine the sound pressure level (SPL) at the audible threshold, it is imperative that the SPL values for each of the attenuator settings on the apparatus be known. It is also imperative that the signal waveform at the transducer faithfully reproduces the input waveform and that the signals are properly timed. The actual process of calibration shall be discussed in detail throughout this text.

Calibration tone: A calibration tone (cal-tone) is frequently used to insure that the experimental apparatus remains in calibration from one test session to another. For example, a 1,000-Hz tone may precede a tape-recorded series of tones or a speech segment. At subsequent test sessions, the level of the tone is adjusted to the same value (using a voltmeter, Vu meter, sound-level meter, or any other appropriate measuring device) as in the previous sessions. This process assures repeatability of the output signal levels of the apparatus.

Center frequency: The center frequency is the frequency at the center of a bandwidth.

Complex tone: A complex tone is a periodic sound wave consisting of a fundamental frequency combined with other sine wave components at different frequencies.

Continuous tone: A continuous tone is a tone which is continuously on.

Coupler: A coupler is a mechanical device which is used to join an earphone to a sound-level meter. The type of coupler most frequently used in the laboratory and clinic contains a volume of precisely 6 cc between the earphone and the microphone diaphragms. This volume approximates the air-space found for an average human ear under an earphone. Thus, the coupler is designed to simulate the impedance characteristics of a normal human ear canal. When a coupler is joined to a microphone on a sound-level meter, it is frequently referred to as an "artificial ear."

Cycle: A cycle consists of the change of a periodic waveform from zero amplitude to a positive peak, to zero, to a negative peak, and back to zero amplitude. The number of cycles occurring in a 1-second interval is the signal frequency.

Decibels: The intensity range over which man is capable of responding to sound has a ratio of about $10^{14}:1$. That is, the power ratio between the absolute threshold and the loudest sound which man can successfully use is about 100 trillion to one. Decibels are logarithmic ratios which compress this extremely large range of intensities into a less unwieldy and more workable system. By definition, decibels for power measures (watts/cm², watts) are defined as:

$$N_{dB} = 10 \log_{10} \frac{I_1}{I_o}$$

where I_1 is an observed power and I_o is a reference power. Decibels for pressures measures (dyne/cm^2, volts, N/m^2, μbars) are defined as:

$$N_{dB} = 20 \log_{10} \frac{P_1}{P_o}$$

where P_1 is an observed pressure and P_o is a reference pressure. Decibels need not only apply to acoustic measures, but may also be extended to any intensive continuum.

Duty cycle: The duty cycle of a device which normally runs in an intermittent mode (alternately on and off) refers to the time the device is operative as compared to the idle time. Duty cycle is generally expressed as a percentage. For example, a 50% duty cycle refers to an equal proportion of on and off periods, whereas a 30% duty cycle refers to an on-interval equaling 30% of the operating time and an off-interval totaling 70% of the operating time.

Dyne: A dyne is the force required to move a mass of 1 gram at a velocity of 1 cm per second.

Dyne per square centimeter (dyne/cm^2): The dyne/cm^2 is a commonly used unit of sound pressure. This unit is equivalent in pressure to 1/1,000,000th of the normal barometric pressure at sea level. Therefore, 1 dyne/cm^2 is equal to 1 μbar and the two units may be interchanged.

Envelope: When observing a waveform on an oscilloscope, it is often advantageous to describe the course of the signal in terms of its maximum instantaneous amplitudes over time. A line passed through these maximum displacement points, both above and below the baseline, is considered to be the envelope of the waveform. For example, in Figure 1.2, the envelope is represented by the *dashed lines.*

Experimental session: An experimental session is the time specified by the experimental design to collect data. Several sessions, each dealing with a different aspect of the design, are frequently used in psychophysical experiments.

Fall-time: The fall-time of an acoustic signal is the time it takes the signal to be reduced from 90% to 10% of its final steady-state value. The effect of fall-time is quite important in psychoacoustic research. A fall-time which is too rapid might bias an experiment dealing with threshold determination because of the introduction of acoustic transients. See Transients and Rise-time.

Flat Response: Flat response is the ability of a device (amplifier, transducer, etc.) to pass all frequencies throughout the audible spectrum in equal proportions. See Frequency response.

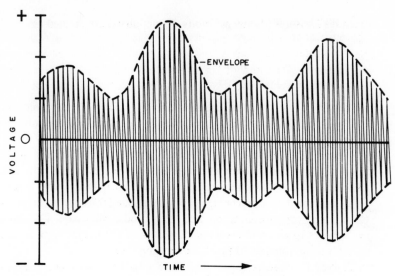

Figure 1.2. Envelope of a waveform.

Flat-spectrum noise: Flat-spectrum noise contains equal energy content for the continuous band of frequencies present in the noise.

Free-field: A free-field is a space filled with a homogeneous medium (e.g., air molecules) whose boundaries do not affect a sound wave which is generated in it. In experimentation, an anechoic chamber is a close approximation of a free field. See Anechoic chamber.

Frequency: The frequency of a pure tone represents the number of complete cycles (Hz) that the sound wave has passed through in a 1-second time period. More generally, frequency refers to the number of recurrences of a periodic phenomenon in a unit of time. The reciprocal of frequency is the period.

Frequency response: The frequency response of a circuit or device is a measure of how efficiently the device (or circuit) passes various frequencies which are applied to it. The frequency response characteristics may be measured by observing the output level of the instrumentation as a function of a constant input level across frequency. For example, the frequency response of an earphone may be measured by applying a constant voltage at the earphone terminals for many frequencies and then measuring the SPL generated by the device for each test frequency. A graph which relates the output level to the input frequency is one example of a frequency response curve.

Frequency response curve: A frequency response curve is a graphic representation of the way a circuit or device responds to various frequencies (of equal input amplitudes) which are applied to it. The ordinate of the function may be expressed in dB SPL, dB re some arbitrary voltage level, voltage, or any other appropriate output measure. The abscissa of the function is frequency. Figure 1.3 shows a response curve for an audiometric earphone (TDH-49). Also shown in the figure is the linear response of the phone, i.e., a graph which relates output SPL to input voltage level.

Fundamental frequency: The fundamental frequency is the lowest frequency component in a complex periodic wave. See Complex tone and Harmonics.

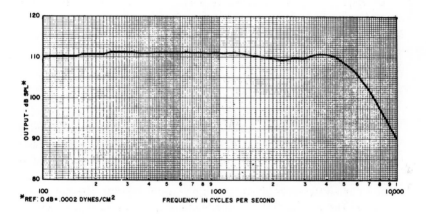

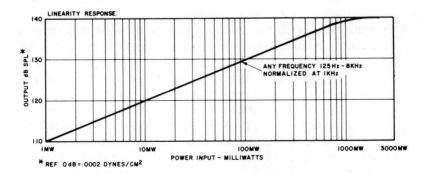

Figure 1.3. Frequency response curve for TDH-49 earphone. Courtesy of ISC/telephonics.

Gain: The gain of an amplifier is a ratio between the input and the output signal levels. Gain may be expressed in terms of voltage or power where the output is divided by the input. More often, however, gain is expressed in dB, with the input power (or voltage) serving as the reference level (I_o or P_o) and the output signal serving as the observed level (I_1 or P_1). See Amplification.

Harmonics: Harmonics are sinusoid components of a complete wave which are exact multiples of the fundamental frequency. The first harmonic is the fundamental frequency itself, while the second and third harmonics are two and three times the fundamental frequency, respectively.

Harmonic distortion: Harmonic distortion is the unwanted introduction of harmonic components of a sine wave input signal which arises as a consequence of the nonlinear response of an amplifier or transducer.

Hertz: Hertz (Hz) is the primary measure of stimulus frequency.

Intensity level: The intensity level in dB of a sound may be determined by the equation:

$$\text{intensity level (IL) in dB} = 10 \log_{10} \frac{I_1}{I_o}$$

where I_1 is a measured intensity in watts/cm^2, and I_o is a reference intensity of 10^{-16} watts/cm^2. This latter value is an approximation of the threshold of hearing at 1,000 Hz for normal hearing young adults.

Intermodulation distortion: Intermodulation distortion is characterized by the presence, at the output of an amplifier, of frequencies equal to the sums and differences of exact multiples of the input frequency components. The presence of intermodulation distortion is caused by nonlinear amplifier response. It should be noted that harmonic components of the input signal are not included as part of the intermodulation distortion. See Harmonic distortion.

Interstimulus interval: The interstimulus interval (ISI) is the time between successive stimulus presentations in an experiment. An example of the ISI is seen in many experiments where the subject is presented with two stimuli and is asked to make some judgment (or adjustment) of the second relative to the first (or vice versa). A subject may be asked to adjust the second stimulus to one-half the apparent pitch of the first stimulus. In this case the ISI would be the time interval between the offset of the first tone (standard) and the onset of the second tone (comparison). In many instances the ISI affects the obtained results, thus necessitating its consideration in the experimental design.

MX-41/AR cushion: The MX-41/AR cushion is commonly mounted on earphones used in experimentation and in audiology clinics. Artificial ears (couplers) are constructed to be used in conjunction with earphones mounted in these cushions. The cushion is doughnut shaped and is made of sponge neoprene. Earphones commonly mounted in these cushions are Telephonics models TDH-39, TDH-49, and TDH-50 and Permoflux models PDR-8 and PDR-10.

Narrow-band noise: Narrow-band noise may be generally defined as a noise whose energy content is restricted to a narrow frequency region. In psychoacoustic experimentation it is often the case that narrow bands of noise are produced by the selective filtering of white-noise. The resultant noise is one of uniform spectrum, but of narrow frequency range. The upper and lower frequency limits of the noise may be defined by its 3 dB down points, i.e., those frequencies where the energy level is 3 dB (half-power) below the average maximum noise amplitude. The difference in Hz between the upper and lower frequency limits of the noise represents the noise bandwidth.

Octave: An octave is a 2:1 or a 1:2 frequency range. For example, 250 Hz and 500 Hz are one octave apart, while the difference between 250 Hz and 1,000 Hz is two octaves.

On-time: The on-time of an acoustic signal is the length of time the signal is presented. If a signal has instantaneous rise- and fall-times, the on-time is simply the time difference between the signal onset and offset. However, the situation is more complex when the stimulus rise- and fall-times are altered. Under these latter conditions various conventions have been adopted which specify the signal duration.

Peak amplitude: Peak amplitude refers to the maximum instantaneous displacement of a waveform from its null point.

Peak clipping: Peak clipping refers to the process whereby a device such as a transducer or amplifier limits its output amplitude as the input signal is increased beyond a certain level. The device output may be linearly related to the input signal up to a given level, but above this point the response becomes nonlinear. Any further increase in the input signal is not reproduced in the output waveform.

Peak-to-peak amplitude: Peak-to-peak amplitude is the sum of the extreme positive and negative excursions of a waveform about its null point.

Period: The period of a periodic event is the time required to complete one cycle. Period may be defined as $1/f$, where f is frequency. Thus, the period of a 1,000-Hz tone is 1/1000 or one one-thousandth of a second.

Phase: The phase of a periodic waveform represents that portion of a cycle which has elapsed at a given instant in time, relative to some arbitrary reference point. The time period required to complete one cycle can be represented as 360° along the time axis because of the mathematical relation between periodic (or simple harmonic) motion and circular functions. Thus, the phase at any point during a cycle may vary between 0° and 360°. Figure 1.4 shows how phase and amplitude of a sine wave are related. Note that the origin (0°) is arbitrarily chosen to be zero amplitude or the baseline level.

Phase angle: See Phase difference.

Phase difference: Phase difference refers to the relative locations of two periodic waveforms at a given instant in time. For example, if two sine waves are of identical frequency and amplitude, but are started one-fourth cycle apart, their phase difference will be 90°. That is, the first sine wave will have reached its maximum amplitude at the moment that the second sine wave begins.

Pink noise: Pink noise is a noise which has equal energy content per octave. Thus, the spectrum of the noise is inversely proportional to the signal frequency, falling off at a rate of 3 dB/octave.

Pure tone: A pure tone is a sound wave which has a definite tonal quality. The waveform of a pure tone is a sine wave. The frequency of a pure tone (in Hertz) corresponds to the number of complete cycles which the sound wave passes through in a 1-second time period.

Random noise: A random noise is a signal whose instantaneous amplitude is determined in a random, and, therefore, unpredictable, manner. It contains no periodic frequency components and its spectrum is continuous. White-noise is a random noise which traverses a wide frequency range. See White-noise.

Repetition rate: Repetition rate is the number of times an event occurs

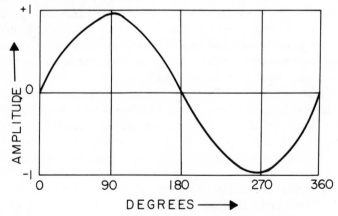

Figure 1.4. Relationship between phase and amplitude of a sine wave.

within a given time period. For example, if a tone pulse is presented once per second, the repetition rate is 1/second.

Rise-time: The rise-time of a signal is the time it takes the signal to rise from 10% to 90% of its final steady value. Figure 1.5 shows the concept of rise-time for a short tone burst. Note that the rise-time in the figure is not instantaneous, but that it occurs gradually over time. If the rise-time were instantaneous an acoustic transient (click) would be clearly audible at the beginning of the tone burst. See Fall-time, Transient.

Root-mean-square amplitude: The root-mean-square amplitude (RMS amplitude) is considered to represent the effective amplitude of an alternating waveform. Specifically, the RMS amplitude is equivalent to the square root of the arithmetical mean of the squares for all the instantaneous amplitudes in the waveform. For the case of a sine wave, the RMS amplitude is equal to the peak amplitude multiplied by 0.707.

Sawtooth wave: A sawtooth wave is periodic in that it is repeated in a definite time interval. The appearance of the wave is sawtooth in nature because the amplitude varies between two values. In general, a longer time interval is required in one direction than in the other. Sawtooth waves are complex waves composed of a fundamental fre-

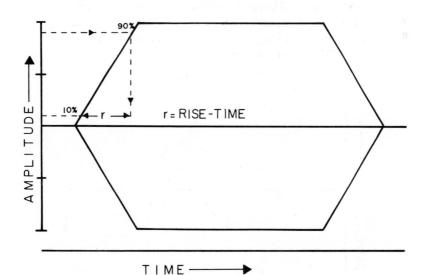

Figure 1.5. Rise-time of a tone burst.

quency and the addition of all the odd and even harmonics of the fundamental. Figure 1.6 shows the general appearance of a sawtooth wave.

Signal-to-noise ratio: A signal-to-noise ratio (S/N ratio) is the ratio between a signal and an ambient or controlled noise. The ratio is generally expressed in dB, and is computed by subtracting the dB value of the noise from the dB value of the signal. For example, an experimenter may be interested in determining the S/N ratio at a subject's threshold for a tone in a white-noise background. If the noise is 60 dB SPL and the tone threshold is 25 dB SPL, the S/N ratio is −35 dB.

Sound field: A sound field is an area which contains sound waves. In the clinic the sound field for tests using loudspeakers is typically a prefabricated booth which is relatively effective in absorbing sound within the closed field and in preventing reflections. Figure 1.7 shows a photograph of a prefabricated audiometric test booth.

Sound-power level: See Watts.

Sound pressure level: Sound pressure level (SPL) in dB may be determined using the expression:

$$N_{dB} = 20 \log_{10} \frac{P_1}{P_o}$$

where P_1 is an observed sound pressure and P_o is an explicitly stated reference pressure. The most commonly used standard reference pressure is 0.0002 dyne/cm^2. This value represents, on the average, the sound pressure at which a normal hearing young adult is first able to hear a 1,000-Hz tone. The standard reference pressure (P_o) may also

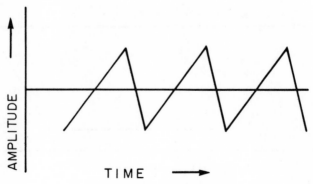

Figure 1.6. Sawtooth waveform.

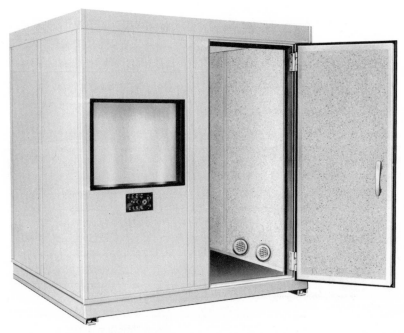

Figure 1.7. Prefabricated audiometric test booth. Courtesy of Industrial Acoustics Company, Inc.

be stated in microbars and newtons per square centimeter (N/cm^2). In the first instance the reference pressure is 0.0002 μbar (1 dyne/cm^2 = 1 μbar). In the second instance the reference pressure is 2×10^{-5} N/m^2 (1 μbar = 0.1 N/m^2).

Spectrum: All acoustic signals may be analyzed into their component frequencies. The results of this process may be plotted as a frequency by amplitude plot known as the signal's spectrum. A *continuous spectrum* is one in which the signal is composed of a continuous and unbroken band of frequencies. On the other hand, a *line spectrum* is one in which the energy content is concentrated at one or more frequencies. Figure 1.8 shows the spectrums of several common types of waveforms.

Spectrum level: The spectrum level of a noise which has a continuous and flat spectrum is defined as the sound pressure level present in each cycle of that noise. The spectrum level may be calculated using the expression:

spectrum level (dB SPL/Hz) =   overall dB SPL of the noise $- 10 \log_{10}$ BW

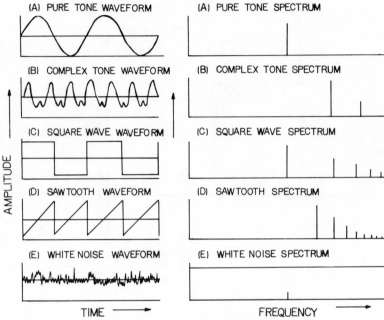

Figure 1.8. Spectrums of common waveforms.

where BW is the bandwidth of the noise in Hertz. For example, if a flat-spectrum noise 2,000 Hz wide has an overall SPL of 70 dB, its spectrum level would be calculated to be $70 - 10 \log_{10} \ 2,000 = 70 - 10 \ (3.3) = 70 - 33.3 = 36.7$ dB SPL/Hz.

Square wave: A square wave is a period wave which alternately assumes two amplitude values for equal time lengths. The transition time between the two levels is negligible, falling in the nanosecond (ns) range (note: 1 ns = one-billionth of a second). Square waves are complex waves composed of a fundamental frequency and (ideally) an infinite series of odd harmonies which decrease in amplitude as their frequency increases. Figure 1.9 shows an ideal square wave.

Standard stimulus: In many psychophysical experiments two signals are presented to a subject for comparison. One signal (usually the first) is called the standard stimulus and the other is called the comparison stimulus. The subject's task is to make some judgment of the comparison relative to the standard. For example, the subject may be asked to judge the loudness of the comparison relative to the loudness of the standard.

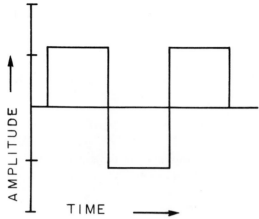

Figure 1.9. Ideal square wave.

TDH-39, TDH-49 earphones: These are earphones commonly used in psychoacoustic experimentation and in the auditory clinic. They are often mounted in MX-41/AR cushions. The frequency response of these earphones is typically limited to about 6,000 Hz.

Transducer: A transducer is a device which converts energy from one form to another. In acoustics the three main types of transducers are earphones (headphones), microphones, and loudspeakers. These devices, of course, convert electrical energy to acoustic energy or vice versa.

Transient: When an acoustic signal is turned on or off rapidly or is presented for a very brief duration, a transient is often produced. In general, a transient may be described as a spreading of the acoustic energy to frequencies other than the test frequency itself. Transients are continuous bands of frequencies whose bandwidths increase as the duration of the acoustic stimulus decreases. To reduce audible transients (which may sound like a click or a thump) infinitely fast rise- and fall-times should be avoided. This may be accomplished by gradually increasing the stimulus amplitude over time. Reduction of transients is quite important in threshold testing since the subject may not respond to the test tone, but to the transient instead.

Watts: Watts are units of power, or the rate at which energy is used. Electrical power in watts is the product of volts multiplied by current. Acoustic power is reported in terms of *sound-power level* (PWL) and may be calculated using the expression:

$$N_{dB} \text{ sound-power level (PWL)} = 10 \log_{10} \frac{W_1}{W_o}$$

where W_1 is an observed power in watts and W_o is a reference power of 10^{-12} watt.

Waveform: The waveform of a signal is the instantaneous amplitude of the signal as a function of time.

Wavelength: The wavelength of a periodic waveform is the distance between corresponding phases of two consecutive cycles. The wavelength in feet may be calculated by the formula:

$$\text{wavelength } (\lambda) = V/f$$

where V is the velocity of sound in air (about 1,080 feet/second) and f is frequency. Thus, the wavelength of a 1,000-Hz tone is 1,080/1,000 or 1.08 feet.

White-noise: White-noise is noise which consists of a continuous spectrum throughout the audible range. Furthermore, the energy per cycle (i.e., spectrum level) is constant for all frequencies. In experimentation, the bandwidth of white-noise may be limited by the frequency response of the transducer used to deliver the signal.

1.2. TERMINOLOGY DEALING WITH
SOME BASIC PSYCHOACOUSTIC PHENOMENA

Absolute Threshold: The absolute threshold is the minimum stimulus intensity which is capable of first eliciting a response. In psychoacoutics the level of the threshold response is often expressed in dB SPL (dB re 0.0002 dyne/cm^2). The absolute threshold is considered to be an average phenomenon. This is because of its tendency to vary as internal and external factors influence the subject. Therefore, the absolute threshold, by convention, is taken to be that stimulus intensity which produces a response half of the time.

Air conduction: Air conduction may be considered to be the normal mode of hearing. That is, the acoustic energy is directed to the inner ear first via the air in the external auditory meatus (ear canal) and then via the transducer action of the middle ear system. The two most common electroacoustic devices used to deliver air-conducted sound to subjects are earphones and loudspeakers.

ANSI (1969): ANSI (1969) refers to a relatively recent standardization of those sound pressure levels which represent audiometric zero for pure tones and for speech. Specifically, ANSI (1969) refers to the American National Standards Institute's *Specification for Audiometers* (ANSI S3.6-1969).

Audiogram: An audiogram is a function which relates the absolute threshold for pure tones in dB hearing threshold level (HTL or dB HL) to stimulus frequency. See Hearing threshold level.

Audiometric zero: Audiometric zero is more frequently referred to as 0 dB HTL or 0 dB HL. It represents the average absolute threshold in dB SPL for a large group of normal hearing individuals. For example, ANSI (1969) standards indicate that audiometric zero at 1,000 Hz is 7 dB SPL, while at 250 Hz audiometric zero is 24.5 dB SPL. (Note that these values were obtained using a TDH-39 earphone mounted in an MX-41/AR cushion.)

Binaural: Listening with two ears.

Bone conduction: Bone conduction is the process whereby acoustic energy reaches the inner ear via the bones in the skull. The transducer used to deliver bone conducted stimuli is called a *bone conduction vibrator.* In routine clinical audiometric testing the vibrator is placed against the mastoid process or forehead with a force of about 200–400 grams. Two principle types of bone conduction have been identified. In *inertial bone conduction,* which is primarily operative at low sound frequencies, the skull is thought to vibrate as one body. The stapes, however, is not rigidly attached to the temporal bone at the oval window. Therefore, when the skull vibrates, both the skull and the stapes will move. However, the stapes will tend to lag behind the movement of the skull because of its resistance to movement (i.e., inertia). The result of this process is the displacment of the stapes in the oval window in much the same manner as in air conduction. In *compression bone conduction,* which occurs at higher sound frequencies, the skull itself is thought to be alternately compressed and expanded as a result of the variations in sound pressure. When the labyrinth is compressed both the oval and round windows bulge since the cochlear fluids are relatively incompressible. However, the round window will expand more because of its greater elasticity. The result of this process is a momentary pressure gradient between the scala tympani and the scala vestibuli, which is an effective stimulus for the hearing mechanism.

Contralateral: Relating to the opposite side.

Critical band: Many psychoacoustic phenomena may be explained using the concept of a critical band. However, the most frequent use of the concept is in masking experiments. Briefly, it is suggested that when a signal (i.e., pure tone) is masked by noise, only those frequency components of the noise which lie in close proximity to the test frequency are influential in the masking process. The noise frequencies which lie outside this critical band surrounding the test frequency do not contribute to the masking process, but merely add to the loudness of the noise. Furthermore, it is suggested that when the tone is just audible in the noise, the energy within the critical band is just equal to that of the tone.

Dichotic listening: Dichotic listening denotes an arrangement where a different auditory stimulus is presented to each ear.

Difference limen: A difference limen (DL) (also known as a differential threshold or a just noticeable difference (JND)) is the smallest increment (or decrement) in a stimulus value that a subject first perceives. The DL is considered to be a statistical value. By convention, it is chosen to be that stimulus value which elicits a response of just being noticeably different 50% of the time. Difference limens may be found for many aspects of the auditory experience. The most frequently found DLs are for stimulus intensity (DL_I) and for frequency (DL_F).

Diotic listening: Diotic listening denotes an arrangement where each ear is presented with an identical auditory stimulus.

Effective masking: The amount of effective masking is numerically equal to the number of decibels (dB) that a given noise shifts the threshold of a second stimulus, usually a tone. For example, a noise which is 10 dB effective will shift a threshold 10 dB, a noise which is 25 dB effective will cause a threshold shift of 25 dB, and so on. The concept of effective masking is based upon the linear relation that exists between masking noise (either wide- or narrow-band) and threshold shift, which occurs after the noise has reached a given intensity level. That is, up to a point masking noise will be ineffective in its masking ability. However, once this level has been passed, there will be a 1:1 correspondance between further masking increments and threshold shift. The point at which the linearity begins is referred to as the *0-dB effective masking level.* It should be noted that the noise level necessary to reach the 0-dB effective masking point varies with stimulus frequency. However, once this point is reached, threshold shift and noise level are linearly related. The effective level (in dB) of a masking noise has been shown to correspond to the sensation level of the critical band about the masked frequency. See Chapter 4.5.

Equal loudness contours: Equal loudness contours (also called isophonic contours) are functions which relate equal loudness sensations (in dB SPL) for different frequency sounds. The reference frequency against which all other frequencies are compared is 1,000 Hz. The *loudness level* of the 1,000 Hz tone is expressed in *phons* and is numerically equal to its SPL (dB re 0.0002 dyne/cm^2). The loudness level (in phons) for any other frequency tone judged to be equally as loud as the 1,000-Hz reference tone is equal to the phon value of the latter. For example, a 60-phon loudness contour would relate the loudness level of a 1,000-Hz tone (at 60 dB SPL) to the SPLs necessary to achieve equal loudness judgments at other sound frequencies across the audible range. See Chapter 4.3.

Fatigue: Auditory fatigue is the difference in decibels (dB) which occurs between absolute threshold measures before and after acoustic stimulation. For example, an experimenter may be interested in knowing the effects of a 10-minute exposure of rock and roll music on the audibility of various frequency test tones. To do this, the experimenter must obtain both pre- and postexposure measures of threshold at each of the frequencies of interest. The difference between these measures is an indication of the auditory fatigue. The interval between the termination of the music (fatiguer) and the postexposure threshold measurement must be explicitly stated as must the level of the music.

Hearing threshold level (hearing level): Hearing threshold level (or hearing level) is expressed as dB HTL or dB HL, respectively. It represents the number of dB relative to audiometric zero at which a subject first perceives a given frequency tone or speech. Thus, 0 dB HTL refers to that SPL which, on the average, is first heard by a group of normal hearing young adults. If a given subject first perceives a stimulus at 50 dB HTL, he or she is considered to have a 50 dB hearing loss. Hearing threshold levels are commonly based upon ANSI (1969) or ISO (1964) standards.

Ipsilateral: Relating to the same side.

ISO (1964): The International Organization for Standardization in 1964 issued standards for audiometric zero for pure tones and speech. ISO standards are similar to the more recent ANSI (1969) standards, except at some of the higher frequencies. Specifically, ISO (1964) refers to ISO/R 389-1964, *Reference Zero for Pure Tone Audiometers.*

Isophonic contour: See Equal loudness contour.

Localization: Localization is the process by which a listener is able to localize sounds in space. Experiments dealing with localization should be performed (ideally) under free field conditions or when the subject is wearing earphones. In the former condition, it is imperative that an anechoic chamber be used to eliminate reflection of the sound off existing surfaces. In the latter condition, the sound may be localized within the head by changing various relations between the stimulation reaching both ears (e.g., intensity, phase, time, etc.).

Loudness: The loudness of a sound is the psychological percept of sound intensity; therefore, the terms *loudness* and *intensity* should not be confused. The difference between loudness and intensity may be best illustrated by noting that when physical intensity (in dB SPL) is doubled (or halved) the difference between the sounds is 6 dB. On the other hand, many psychoacoustic investigations have shown that when loudness is doubled or halved there is, on the average, about a 10-dB difference between the two sounds. Thus, the human ear does not judge loudness on a purely physical basis. Hence, the dichotomy between loudness and intensity must be observed.

Loudness level: The loudness level (in phons) of any frequency tone is equivalent to the sound pressure level (dB re 0.0002 dyne/cm^2) of a 1,000-Hz tone judged to be of equal loudness. For example, a 100-Hz tone may have to be adjusted to a level of about 70 dB SPL in order to equal the loudness of a 1,000-Hz tone at a level of 60 phons (60 dB SPL). Although the SPL of the 100-Hz tone differs from that of the 1,000-Hz tone, both tones have equivalent loudness levels (60 phons). See Equal loudness contour.

Masked threshold: A masked threshold is the threshold for a given stimulus obtained in the presence of a masker. The masked threshold may be expressed in dB SPL, dB HTL, or any other appropriate intensive measure.

Masking: Masking refers to the number of decibels (dB) that one sound (masker) raises the audible threshold for another sound (signal). Maskers may be any type of auditory stimulus. However, in psychoacoustics and audiology the most frequently used maskers are white-noise, narrow-band noise, and pure tones. In audiology, masking noise is used to raise the threshold of the nontest ear in order to eliminate cross-hearing. The term *threshold shift* is used frequently to describe the masking influence of one stimulus upon the audibility of another.

Mel: The mel is an arbitrary unit used in the scaling of pitch sensation. A value of 1,000 mels equals the apparent pitch of a 1,000-Hz tone set to a loudness level of 55 phons (55 dB SPL). See Pitch and Chapter 4.3.

Monaural listening: Monaural listening is listening with one ear only.

Phon: The phon is the unit of loudness level. The number of phons for any frequency tone is numerically equal to the dB SPL of a 1,000-Hz tone judged to be equally loud. See Equal loudness contour and Loudness level.

Pitch: The pitch of a tone represents the psychological percept of frequency, and the two terms should not be confused. *Pitch is perceptual* while *frequency is physical.* An example of the dichotomy which exists between pitch and frequency may best be seen in the psycho-physical scale which relates these two attributes, the mel scale. The mel scale shows clearly that when the pitch of a tone is doubled (or halved) the judged frequency is not what would be expected on a purely physical basis. Furthermore, the mel scale shows that pitch and frequency cannot be related in any simple manner. See Mel and Chapter 4.3.

Psychophysical scales: Psychophysical scales are functions which relate subjective sensations to physical continua. That is, they are designed to indicate functional relationships between the magnitude of sensory sensations and physical magnitude. The most advanced psychophysical scales, ratio scales, are designed so that they preserve information about ratios between sensations. Ratio scaling methods have been used extensively in establishing the relations between loudness and intensity and pitch and frequency. See Loudness, Pitch, and Chapter 4.3.

Sensation level: The sensation level of a sound (expressed as dB SL) represents the number of decibels that the sound is above the audible threshold. For example, if a subject's threshold for a tone is 10 dB SPL, a tone at 75 dB SPL would be 65 dB SL. It should be noted that dB SL *always* refers to the level above threshold for *one individual only,* whereas dB HTL (HL) refers to an individual's threshold relative to established norms (e.g., ANSI or ISO). See Hearing threshold level.

Sone: The sone is an arbitrary unit of loudness sensation. By definition, 1 sone is equivalent to the loudness of a 1,000-Hz tone at a level of 40 dB SL. See Chapter 4.3.

Temporal summation (integration): Temporal summation (or temporal integration) refers to the functional relationship which exists between auditory intensive responses and the duration of acoustic stimuli. The temporal summation process has been extensively investigated at the audible threshold and at suprathreshold levels (i.e., temporal summation of loudness). See Chapter 4.4.

Threshold shift: Threshold shift in decibels (dB) is equal to the difference in the threshold level of an unmasked stimulus and the threshold for the same stimulus in the presence of a masker. For example, if a tone has an unmasked threshold level of 15 dB SPL and a masked threshold level of 45 dB SPL, the threshold shift is 30 dB. See Masked threshold.

chapter 2

BASIC INSTRUMENTATION FOR PSYCHOACOUSTICS

The rapid growth of contemporary research in psychoacoustics and audiology is directly related to the availability of electronic instrumentation. Without the precision of stimulus control and measurement afforded by electronic instrumentation, research in the field would be severely limited. If any science is to flourish, it is requisite that the procedures and measurement techniques used in one laboratory be duplicated at other locations. Fortunately, contemporary instrumentation gives the researcher the opportunity to scrutinize results obtained at other laboratories and to have his own work scrutinized.

When entering a psychoacoustic/audiological research laboratory for the first time, one is often overwhelmed by the plethora of wires, cables, knobs, and instruments. This situation, however, is not as complicated as it may at first appear. A basic laboratory contains instruments which may generally be separated into five categories according to their function. Table 2.1 lists each of these categories as well as some of the basic instruments found within each. The category listings in Table 2.1 represent a logical sequence for the arrangement of the various circuit components in many psychoacoustic investigations. This, however, will become more apparent throughout the text.

2.1. PRIMARY SIGNAL SOURCES

The primary signal in a psychoacoustic investigation is that stimulus (or stimuli) which is to serve as the independent variable in the study. That is, it is that stimulus which is directly under the experimenter's control and

Table 2.1. Basic psychoacoustic instrumentation categories

Primary signal sources	Signal shapers	Intercategory units	Output transducers	Monitoring and measurement instruments
AF oscillators	Electronic switches	Impedance matching transformers	Earphones	AC voltmeters
Function generators	Attenuators	Mixing networks	Microphones	Oscilloscopes
Noise generators	Filters			Sound-level meters
Microphones	Amplifiers			Wave analyzers
Magnetic tape recorders				Graphic level recorders
				Tape recorders
				Counters

which will elicit the desired response (dependent variable). The majority of experiments in the field utilize either pure tones, noise, or speech as the primary signals. For example, when determining an absolute threshold for tones the primary signal is, of course, a pure tone which is generated by an audio frequency (AF) oscillator. However, if the experimenter desires to determine the effects of white-noise on the absolute threshold of the tone, both the masking noise and the pure tone serve as the primary signals.

Audio Frequency (AF) Oscillators

The audio frequency oscillator is the most basic instrument in audiometric and psychoacoustic research. Nearly every classical area of auditory experimentation is dependent upon the use of AF oscillators. These oscillators provide sine wave outputs which are continuously variable in frequency throughout the auditory range (20–20,000 Hz) and somewhat beyond. Furthermore, the output voltages from these oscillators must remain relatively unchanged for a given gain (intensity) setting over the entire frequency range.

Two types of audio frequency oscillators are commonly used in the laboratory and clinic. The first, and most common, is the R-C (Wien-bridge) oscillator. In a laboratory tube-type R-C oscillator which contains two tubes (such as that seen in Figure 2.1), oscillation is caused by positive feedback from the plate of the second tube to the grid of the first tube. The frequency of the oscillator is varied by changing either the resistive (R) or capacitive (C) elements in the feedback network, which is arranged in a Wien–bridge. In general, tuning of these oscillators is accomplished using a variable air capacitor, whereas bandswitching is accomplished by switching resistances.

A characteristic feature of many R-C type laboratory oscillators, which the reader unfamiliar with oscillators may use in their identification, is that they cover approximately one decade (10:1 ratio) of frequency for one rotation of the main frequency dial. Thus, the audible spectrum is traversed by overlapping frequency sweeps which are controlled by the oscillator main frequency dial and by an associated range switch. The range switch is often arranged so that the output frequencies are X 1, X 10, X 100, or X 1,000 the value indicated on the main frequency dial.

The second type of audio frequency oscillator found in the laboratory is the beat frequency, or heterodyne oscillator. The principle advantage of beat frequency oscillators (BFOs) is that they traverse a large frequency range with only a single rotation of the main frequency dial. Thus, the need for bandswitching, as with R-C oscillators, is reduced. Beat frequency oscillators typically use two high frequency oscillating circuits to achieve their audio frequency outputs. The first oscillating circuit provides a fixed

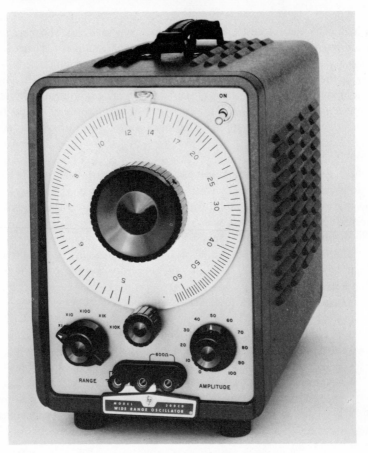

Figure 2.1. Photograph of a laboratory R-C oscillator (Hewlett-Packard 200 CD) using a Wien-Bridge feedback circuit. Courtesy of Hewlett-Packard.

frequency, while the second circuit may be varied in frequency. The outputs of the two circuits are electronically mixed, and a difference frequency is obtained. For example, the fixed frequency oscillator may be set to 100 kHz, while the variable oscillator may range between 100 kHz and 120 kHz. The difference tones will now lie within the audio frequency range (0–20 kHz). It should be noted that the two high frequency oscillators used to produce the difference tone should be extremely stable because a small percentage frequency drift at these high frequencies will cause a relatively large frequency shift in the resultant audio frequency output.

Audio frequency oscillators not only provide the primary signal source for psychoacoustic and audiological investigations, but are also extensively used in the calibration of individual circuit components and apparatus arrangements.

Function Generators

Function generators are instruments that provide a choice of different waveforms in addition to sine waves. That is, in addition to the production of conventional sine waves, these generators may also produce square waves, sawtooth waves, triangular waves, and pulses. The repetition rate (frequency) of these waveforms is variable over a wide frequency range. Function generators serve many purposes in research and in determining the operating characteristics of instrumentation. For example, square waves may be used to check the frequency response of amplifiers. This is accomplished by applying a square-wave signal to the input of the amplifier and then observing the output waveform with an oscilloscope. If the amplifier frequency response is not uniform across frequency, the shape of the output waveform will differ somewhat from that of the input waveform. The manner in which the output differs from the input serves as an indicator of the amplifier frequency response. Figure 2.2 shows a function generator (Heath/Schlumberger EU-81A) which provides triangular, sine, and square waves. The frequency of these waveforms is variable over seven decades from 0.1 Hz to 1 MHz.

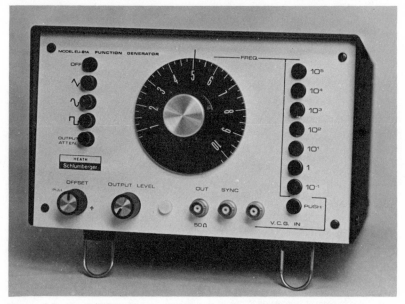

Figure 2.2. Heath/Schlumberger EU-81A function generator which provides sine, square, and triangular waveforms.

Random Noise Generators

Random noise generators also represent one of the most basic primary signal sources in clinical audiology and psychoacoustic research. Random noise has been used extensively in studies dealing with masking and critical band determination, scaling, temporal summation, and the perception of speech in noise. In the auditory clinic, random noise is routinely applied to the nontest ear to eliminate cross-hearing.

Most general purpose random noise generators provide a noise source whose instantaneous amplitudes are random and are, therefore, unpredictable. These instantaneous amplitudes, however, are distributed in a normal or gaussian manner. Furthermore, the noise signals are of uniform (flat) spectrum in the frequency range between about 20 and 20,000 Hz, and frequently beyond. Random noise of uniform spectrum over a wide frequency range is, of course, referred to as white-noise. Random noise may be selectively filtered to provide bands of noise of specified bandwidth (e.g., 1 octave or $^1/_3$ octave), or the noise may be shaped as in the generation of pink noise.

Figure 2.3 shows a random noise generator (General Radio 1390-B) which provides three uniform noise spectra (20—20 kHz, 20—500 kHz, and

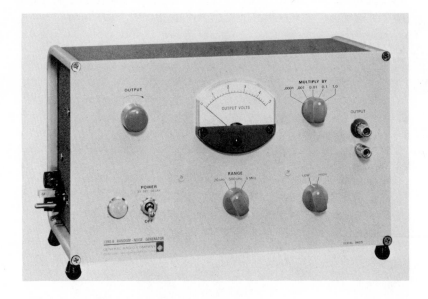

Figure 2.3. Random noise generator (General Radio 1390-B) providing three uniform noise spectra. Courtesy of General Radio.

20–5 MHz). The level of the noise may be monitored using a built-in monitoring meter.

Microphones

Microphones may also serve to provide a primary signal. In general, a microphone is an electroacoustic transducer which converts sound energy into electrical energy. There are a number of different types of microphones, each with its own characteristics. The following provides a brief description of the operating principles of some common microphone types.

The operating principle of *carbon microphones* is illustrated in Figure 2.4. It is seen that the active element is a hollow button which is filled with carbon granules. A battery is placed in series with the button so that any current flow in the battery must also flow through the granules. A diaphragm is rigidly coupled to one side of the button. When sound pressure impinges itself upon the diaphragm, the mechanical pressure placed upon the carbon granules changes in response to the alternating pressures. These changes, in turn, cause the resistance of the carbon button to change, thereby causing the current in the circuit to change in the same manner. The end-product of this process is an alternating current which has the same characteristics as the original sound source.

The principal advantages of carbon microphones are that they are: 1) sensitive, 2) able to generate a relatively high output voltage, and 3) relatively inexpensive. Their principal disadvantages are: 1) a limited frequency response (generally confined to 3,000 Hz and below and 2) the

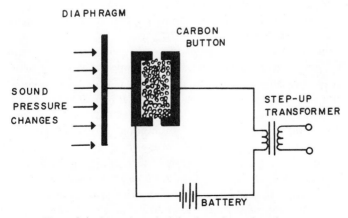

Figure 2.4. Operating principle of a carbon microphone.

presence of an annoying hiss because of the ever present current flow through the carbon button.

The *crystal* (or *piezoelectric*) *microphone* is the simplest of the types to be discussed here. The active element is a crystal (usually Rochelle salt). Rochelle salt, like other crystalline substances, when deformed by mechanical pressure, generates an electrical potential between its opposite surfaces. Therefore, in one type of crystal microphone, a diaphragm is rigidly connected to one surface of the crystal. Sound pressures applied to the diaphragm cause the diaphragm to move. This, in turn, causes slight deformations of the crystalline slab which then cause a potential to be generated. The potential varies in direct proportion to the sound pressure changes, and represents the microphone output.

The primary advantages of crystal microphones are that they generate a relatively high voltage output and that their frequency response (about 50–8,000 Hz) is considerably greater than that of carbon microphones. The impedance of a crystal microphone is high enough so that impedance matching is not necessary between the microphone and an amplifier input. The primary disadvantages of crystal microphones are their susceptibility to changes caused by heat and moisture and their liability to mechanical shock.

Electrodynamic (or *dynamic*) *microphones* are constructed in much the same manner as dynamic earphones and speakers. A small coil is cemented to the diaphragm. The coil, in turn, is placed in the field of a permanent magnet. When the diaphragm vibrates in response to acoustic energy, the coil also moves back and forth. This action induces an alternating voltage in the coil which is directly proportional to the original sound source. The frequency response of dynamic microphones is flat to about 8,000 Hz, and the response mode is generally omnidirectional (e.g., equally responsive in all directions).

A *ribbon* (or *velocity*) *microphone* is constructed so that a corregated metallic ribbon is suspended between the poles of a strong permanent magnet. When sound waves strike the ribbon, it vibrates, thus cutting the magnetic field. This cutting action then induces an alternating voltage in the ribbon which corresponds to the signal characteristics. The frequency response of ribbon microphones is from about 30–12,000 Hz. The construction of these microphones, however, gives them a bidirectional response mode with maximum sensitivity in the front and back directions.

Condenser (or *electrostatic*) *microphones* are used extensively for precise measurements and for calibration. This is because of their wide frequency response (which may extend over the entire audio range), their high sensitivity, and their stability over time. Condenser microphones derive their name because they are, in fact, small condensers. These microphones are constructed of two thin metallic plates which are in close proximity to each other. While one plate is fixed in position, the other is moveable and serves as the diaphragm. These two plates then serve as electrodes of a capacitor. The diaphragm (or membrane) is attached to the microphone housing, which serves as the ground. The fixed plate (polarization electrode or back plate) is isolated from the housing by an insulator such as quartz. A DC polarization voltage is maintained between the plates. When a sound wave causes the diaphragm to vibrate, the capacitance between the plates changes. The resultant is the generation of an AC voltage across a load resistor. This alternating voltage serves as the output of the microphone. The response mode of a condenser microphone is omnidirectional. Figure 2.5 shows a cross-sectional view of a typical condenser microphone.

Magnetic Tape Recorders

Magnetic tape recorders are often used to provide the primary signal source, particularly when the signal is of a complex nature and must remain unaltered among sessions. When the recording method is used, the original signal is first stored on magnetic tape. At a later time the prerecorded stimuli are played through the experimental system. The principle advantage of tape-recorded stimuli is, of course, the uniformity of stimulus presentation from one test session to another and from one individual to another. The reader is referred to the Monitoring and Measurement Instruments section of the present chapter for a more complete description of the magnetic tape recording process.

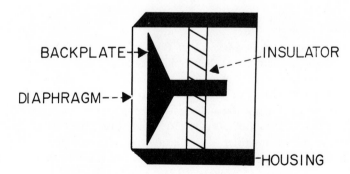

Figure 2.5. Cross-section of a condenser microphone.

2.2. SIGNAL SHAPERS

Signal shapers are instruments that alter the primary signal in some fashion.

Attenuators

Attenuators shape the signal by reducing its intensity. Attenuators used in the laboratory and clinic are frequently calibrated in one or multiple decibel steps which may extend up to a total range of 110 dB. That is, the output voltage from a primary signal source may be applied to the input terminals of an attenuator, and then may be reduced in precise dB steps using the attenuator controls. The output level of any transducer (e.g., earphone) which follows the attenuator in the circuit will then be reduced by an equivalent dB value. For example, in a simple circuit which consists of an oscillator, attenuator, and an earphone (of equivalent impedance values), a voltage of, for example, 0.5 volt may produce 100 dB SPL at the earphone with 0-dB attenuation present. If 20-dB attenuation is then introduced, the voltage at the attenuator output will drop to one-tenth (20 dB) of the voltage present at the attenuator input, thereby reducing the output SPL to 80 dB.

Attenuators are electronically designed so that they present a constant load to the amplifier (or other device) which precedes them in the circuit. Thus, the operating characteristics of the preceding device remain unaffected by the presence of the attenuator, and only the attenuator output is varied. Attenuators are also designed to have a very wide frequency response.

Figure 2.6 shows a laboratory-type attenuator (Hewlett-Packard 350D) which is variable in 1-dB steps to a total of 110 dB. Note that one control reduces the input voltage by 1-dB steps and the other control by decade (10-dB) steps.

Amplifiers

Amplifiers are signal shapers in that they increase the signal applied to them. Although there are a considerable number of amplifier types (e.g., differential amplifiers, DC amplifiers, and tuned amplifiers among others), the present text is limited to general-purpose, untuned audio frequency amplifiers which traverse the audio frequency spectrum and perhaps somewhat beyond. These amplifiers may serve to increase either voltage, power, or both. A voltage amplifier of the untuned type (also called a preamplifier) is frequently used to increase low signal levels from transducers (or another signal source) to a level sufficiently high enough to be used by a

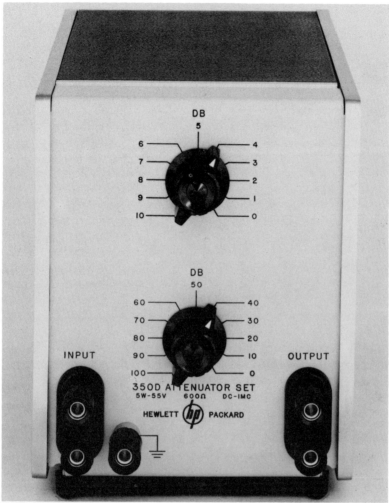

Figure 2.6. Variable attenuator (Hewlett-Packard 350D) which covers a 110-dB range. Courtesy of Hewlett-Packard.

power amplifier. For example, microphones often produce low level signal outputs. To boost the signal strength, the microphone output may first be led to the input of a preamplifier. The output from the preamplifier then serves as the input for subsequent power amplification. An audio frequency power amplifier is designed to drive one or more output transducers with a minimum amount of signal distortion. It is often the case, however, that a single unit will contain both voltage and power amplification stages, thus eliminating the need for separate units.

Filters

Filters are signal shapers which limit the frequency response characteristics of the primary signal source. Filters may be classified as low-pass, high-pass, band-pass, and band-reject, according to their function. Low-pass filters are units which pass frequencies below an adjusted cut-off frequency and attenuate frequencies above this point, High-pass filters pass only frequencies higher than an adjusted cut-off frequency, while attenuating frequencies below that point. Band-pass filters pass only those frequencies in a specified bandwidth while attenuating frequencies outside the band. On the other hand, band-reject filters attenuate a band of frequencies and pass frequencies both above and below this band. For all filter modes the band limits (or cut-off frequency in the cases of either high- or low-passed signals) are taken as that point(s) where the filter response is 3 dB below the average level of the passband. Furthermore, the filter roll-off or attenuation rate is specified in dB/octave.

Figure 2.7 shows a variable filter unit (Rockland 432) which may be used in each of the four filter modes discussed above. In general, this unit consists of two identical filter channels. Each channel has separate input and output terminals, and has both high- and low-pass filter functions. The channels may be used in series (as in the high-, low-, and band-pass modes) or in parallel (as in the band-reject mode). The filter sections may be cascaded to provide considerably greater attenuation rates in the high- and low-pass modes. (To cascade filters is to use the output of one filter as the input to a second filter. Both filters are set in the same mode of operation and both have identical cut-off frequencies.) The attenuation rate for one section alone is about 24 dB/octave. When the two sections are cascaded, the attenuation rate is increased to 48 dB/octave.

Electronic Switches

Electronic switches are signal shapers which serve to turn audio signals on and off with precise rise and fall characteristics. The use of electronic switches in hearing research is particularly important in the areas of threshold determination and in the study of temporal phenomena. This is based upon the fact that, when an acoustic signal is switched on or off abruptly, transient sound energy is produced which may serve to bias the experimental results. To reduce the possibility of transient distortion, infinitely fast rise- and fall-times are avoided. This is often accomplished using electronic switches which are adjusted so that the signal rise- and

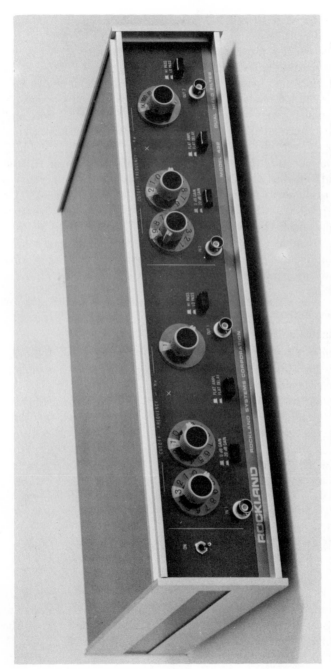

Figure 2.7. Variable filter unit (Rockland 432) which may be used in four filter modes. Courtesy of Rockland Systems Corporation.

fall-times are between 10 and 100 msec, depending upon the total duration of the test signal.

Electronic switches may be timed by internal circuitry or by external
control from separate interval timers or manual switches. To illustrate, the
Allison 408 electronic switch module may be operated in any of four
stimulus presentation modes. (The chosen mode is, of course, primarily
dependent upon the experimental design.) In the first mode, "auto-on,"
the electronic switch alternately presents each of its two channels (A and
B) continuously, with the signal durations and rise- and fall-times of both
channels being identical. In the second mode, "auto-off," a manual lever
switch (A or B) is used to present as many presentations of either time A
or B pulses as the experimenter desires. In the third mode, "manual," the
experimenter may manually present the signal in either channel for as long
as the switch is held. The fourth mode, "remote," is identical to the third
mode except that the signals may be controlled from a position remote
from the main module. Again, as in the third mode, the rise- and fall-time
controls on the main module remain operative.

2.3. INTERCATEGORY DEVICES

Impedance-matching Transformers

When instruments are interconnected in an experimental circuit, it is often
the case that the output impedance of one instrument is not the same as
the input impedance of the following instrument. (Impedance (Z) is the
total opposition to the flow of alternating current from one instrument
(or circuit) to another. It is measured in ohms (Ω)). In order that there
may be a maximum transfer of energy between the instruments, the input
impedance of the second instrument (load) should equal the output
impedance of the first instrument (generator). To achieve this, a matching
transformer is interposed between the two. These transformers, through
wire turns ratios between their primary and secondary coils, are able to
match the load impedance to that of the generator, thus effecting the
maximum power transfer.

In the ideal transformer, the following relation holds true:

$$Z_p = N^2 Z_s.$$

In this equation, Z_p is the impedance looking into the transformer primary
from the generator, Z_s is the impedance of the load which is connected to
the transformer secondary, and N is the transformer turns ratio. The
equation states, in effect, that the secondary load impedance may be
transformed to a different value which appears across the primary termi-

nals of the transformer. By choosing the appropriate turns ratio, the impedance across the primary terminals may be set to match the specific value required for optimal operation of the generator. To determine the proper turns ratio the following equation may be used:

$$N = \sqrt{\frac{Z_p}{Z_s}}.$$

This equation, of course, is simply a restatement of the previous equation, but solved for N. For example, if an amplifier which requires a 600-Ω load for optimal performance is connected to a 10-Ω earphone via a matching transformer, the turns ratio should be:

$$N = \sqrt{\frac{600}{10}} = 60 = 7.75.$$

That is, the primary windings should have 7.75 times the number of turns as the secondary windings.

Mixing Networks

Mixing networks are used when two signal sources are to be applied to a common input point. For example, if an experiment is designed to investigate the relation between speech discrimination and the level of white-noise, both the speech and noise signals would have to be combined. If these sources were directly connected, however, the possibility of one circuit affecting the other would be present. Therefore, to isolate one circuit from the other and still obtain a combined output, a resistive mixing network is used. These networks may also be used in reverse to split a single input into two separate branches. Figure 2.8 shows a simple resistive mixing (or splitting) network. Note that both source impedances and the load impedance are of equal values. Also note that the four resistors have the same value. This latter value is equal to the common source or load impedance. For example, if the source and load values are all 10 ohms, the resistor values should be 10 ohms.

2.4. OUTPUT TRANSDUCERS

Without suitable output transducers to convert electrical energy to acoustic energy, psychoacoustic research and clinical audiology would be severely limited. Fortunately, contemporary design of both earphones and loudspeakers is such that the electrical signals may be faithfully reproduced without the introduction of appreciable distortion or transients.

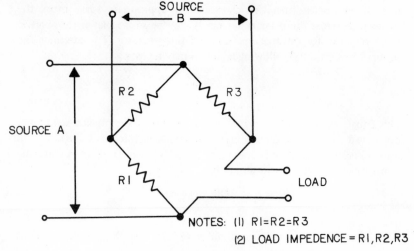

Figure 2.8. Resistive mixing and splitting network.

Earphones

Earphones are output transducers which are designed to be worn against the ears, either singly or in pairs. There are a number of different operating principles of earphones which closely parallel those seen earlier for microphone operation.

Crystal earphones utilize the piezoelectrical properties of certain crystals such as Rochelle salt. In these earphones the diaphragm is caused to move as a result of the deformations caused in the material by the introduction of audio frequency currents to electrodes attached to the crystal slab.

Magnetic earphones consist of a metal diaphragm which is in close proximity to a permanent magnet. The magnet is surrounded by a coil of fine wire. When audio frequency currents are sent through the wire coil, the magnetic field alternately increases and decreases. This, in turn, causes the diaphragm to move in and out in accordance with the field changes.

Electrostatic earphones are based upon the same operating principle as electrostatic (condenser) microphones, but in reverse. That is, these earphones are constructed of two thin conductive surfaces which face each other, and serve as the electrodes of a condenser. One surface is rigid while the other is flexible. The latter surface serves as the diaphragm. To operate, an incoming audio frequency current must first be converted to a

DC polarizing current. This DC polarizing voltage, when applied between the two electrode surfaces, results in movement of the diaphragm. The movement then serves to produce the sound wave.

Dynamic earphones are the most frequently used earphones in both the laboratory and clinic. The working principle is identical to that of conventional permanent magnet loudspeakers (to be discussed). A small coil of wire (voice coil) is rigidly fastened to a nonmetallic membrane which serves as the diaphragm. The coil is placed near a permanent magnet. When audio frequency current is applied to the coil, magnetic fields are induced which cause the coil to be either attracted or repelled from the magnet. As the coil moves back and forth, it moves the diaphragm which is attached to it. This, of course, then causes the air molecules to be alternately compressed and rarefied.

The primary advantage of using earphones as output transducers is that they afford excellent control of the sound levels which reach the subject's ears. Furthermore, the intensities to both ears may be controlled independently.

Loudspeakers

Loudspeakers used in psychoacoustics are almost always of the permanent magnet (PM) dynamic variety. They are constructed of three basic parts. The first is a strong permanent magnet which is often of the Alnico type. (Alnico magnets are capable of great magnetic retentivity. They derive their name from the alloy used in their manufacture—aluminum, nickle, cobalt plus iron.) The second part, the voice coil, consists of a number of wire turns wound about a circular form and then suspended around the permanent magnet. The third part is the cone. The cone is attached to the voice coil. It is generally conical in shape and is constructed of light cardboard. The cone is attached to the loudspeaker superstructure at its outer perimeter.

The operating principle of PM loudspeakers is the same as that for dynamic earphones. When audio frequency current flows through the voice coil, the voice coil becomes an electromagnet. The magnetic field of the voice coil then interacts with the permanent magnetic field. This interaction takes the form of alternating attractions and repulsions which causes the voice coil to move. Since the cone is firmly attached to the voice coil, it also moves. The movement of the cone then causes the air molecules to be displaced. Figure 2.9 shows a cross-sectional view of a typical PM loudspeaker.

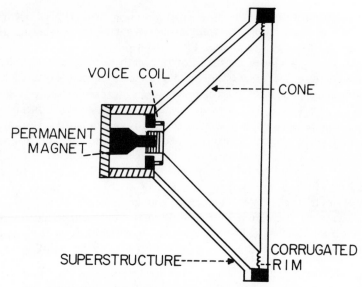

Figure 2.9. Cross-sectional view of a permanent magnet loudspeaker.

2.5. MONITORING AND MEASUREMENT INSTRUMENTS

Monitoring and measurement instruments, although integral parts of experimental circuits are, in fact, independent of these circuits. That is, those
instruments which are electrically connected to the apparatus have such
high input impedances that a minimum amount of current is drawn from
the signal sources. Other instruments, such as sound-level meters, are
mechanically coupled to the experimental apparatus and, therefore, do not
affect the circuit's electrical operation.

AC Voltmeters

AC voltmeters are probably the most commonly used measurement and
monitoring instruments in the laboratory. These instruments are capable
of reading extremely low AC voltages, as commonly encountered in
psychoacoustic research. Although their functions are identical, these
instruments are known by several different names depending upon their
internal component structure. The vacuum-tube AC voltmeter is known as
a VTVM. If the instrument is primarily composed of transistors, it may be
known as a TVM. A DVM, on the other hand, is a voltmeter of the digital
readout variety.

Analog (meter-type) AC voltmeters typically have meter scales which
are calibrated in both voltage and decibels. The arrangement of these two

complementary scales may differ depending upon the design of the individual instrument. In the first and most common form, the voltage scale values are linear, while the dB scale is logarithmic. The range switches on instruments calibrated in this fashion are typically arranged in a 1–3–10 sequence. That is, they may start with a value of 1 millivolt full scale, and then full scale values of 3, 10, 30, 100, 300, 1,000 (1 volt), 3 volts, and so on up to much higher voltages. Voltage on these instruments is read from two separate scales which are arranged so that the difference between the scales is 10 dB (a voltage ratio of 3.16). The decibel scale on these meters typically has a reference point (0 dB) set at a voltage of 0.775 volt on the 1-volt (1,000 millivolt) range. This reference point is 0 dBm, a commonly used reference in audio work. By convention, 0 dBm represents 1 milliwatt (0.01 watt) of power across a 600-ohm load. Since Ohms' law states that

$$\text{voltage } (E) = \sqrt{\text{power } (W) \times \text{resistance } (R)},$$

then the equation solved for E is 0.775 volt. Decibel measurements may be read with reference to 0 dBm if measured across a 600-ohm load (only) or one voltage may be related to another in dB for any other constant impedance load. Figures 2.10a and 2.10b show two laboratory-type AC meters (Hewlett-Packard 400 H and Ballantine 3045A) which employ linear voltage scales and logarithmic dB scales.

The second type of meter face arrangement is found on instruments that respond logarithmically to the applied voltage values. In these instruments, the voltage scale is logarithmic, while the dB scale is linear. The range switch on these instruments often covers 20 dB or a 10:1 voltage ratio. This is considerably larger than the 10 dB (3.16 voltage ratio) covered by the previously described instruments. Thus, the need for switching ranges using these latter instruments is considerably reduced. Figure 2.11 shows a logarithmically responding AC voltmeter (Ballantine 3056A). Note that the range switch is arranged in decades and that the bottom of the voltage scale does not have a 0-volt value, but rather a value of 1. It is, therefore, to be expected that the pointer will rest to the left of the calibrated values when the instrument is not in use. A primary difference between logarithmic and linear responding voltmeters is that the former instruments are equally accurate over their entire scale, whereas linearly responding units are most accurate only at the upper ends of their scales.

AC voltmeters may generally be classified into one of three types. The first and most common type responds to the average (full-wave rectified) value of the incoming voltage at each and every point along the waveform. For a sine wave the average value corresponds to 0.636 times the peak voltage. Thus, calibration of these meters in terms of RMS volts (the

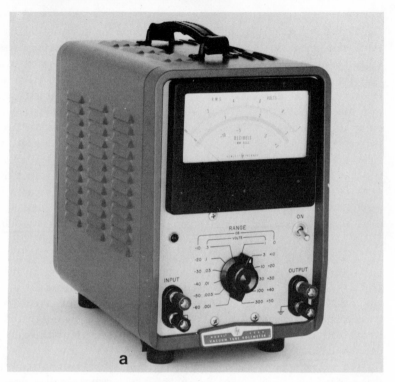

Figure 2.10a. Hewlett-Packard 400H AC voltmeter. Courtesy of Hewlett-Packard.

universally accepted voltage measure) for sinusoids simply requires multiplication by a constant value of 1.11. (The RMS value of a sinusoid is 0.707 times the peak value. Therefore, 0.707/0.636 = 1.11.) The reader should bear in mind, however, that the use of these average-responding meters will only provide the correct RMS value for sine wave signals. The voltage readings will not be true RMS values for other waveforms. The two AC voltmeters seen in Figure 2.10 are average-responding instruments.

Peak-responding voltmeters are also calibrated in terms of RMS volts. For sine wave signals these meters read 0.707 times the peak voltage value and, therefore, require no further multiplication constants as do the average-responding meters. However, like the average-responding meters, any waveform other than a sinusoid will not yield a true RMS value.

True RMS-responding voltmeters have been developed. These instruments will indicate the true effective value of complex waveforms as well as simple sinusoids.

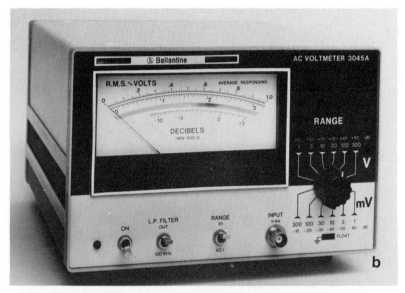

Figure 2.10*b*. Ballantine 3045A AC voltmeter. Courtesy of Ballantine Laboratories.

Oscilloscopes

The oscilloscope is an almost indispensable instrument in the psychoacoustic laboratory. Its functions are varied and may include the following uses: 1) signal waveform analysis, 2) voltage measurements, 3) duration measurements, 4) phase measurements, 5) frequency measurements, 6) input vs. output waveform comparisons, and 7) frequency response measurements.

In general, an oscilloscope is an instrument which provides a visual display (on the phosphorescent coating of a cathode-ray tube) of the instantaneous voltages of signals as a function of time. The visual display is usually represented in terms of X and Y coordinates. The X axis represents time, whereas the Y axis represents the voltage amplitude of the input signal. The greater the input voltage, the greater the Y axis deflection.

An oscilloscope consists of three basic sections exclusive of the common power supply. These include: the cathode-ray tube, the time base generator, and the vertical deflection amplifier.

The cathode-ray tube (CRT) is the heart of an oscilloscope. In the neck of the CRT is an electron gun which shoots a narrow beam of electrons to the phosphor-coated face of the tube. When the electron beam strikes the phosphor coating, the phosphor fluoresces (glows) in a single spot only. To produce movement of the electron beam the tube is constructed so that, as

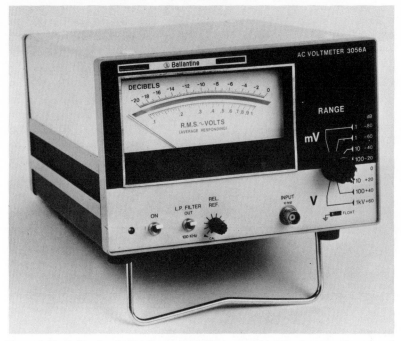

Figure 2.11. Ballantine 3065A logarithmically responding AC voltmeter. Courtesy of
Ballantine Laboratories.

soon as the beam leaves the gun, it passes through two pairs of deflection
plates. The first pair produces horizontal deflection, while the second pair
produces vertical deflection of the beam. Movement in either direction is
the result of electrostatic deflection caused by appropriate voltages to the
plates. Since electrons are negatively charged particles, they will be attracted to a positively charged plate and repelled by a negatively charged
plate. Therefore, if the beam is to be bent down, a negative potential
should be present at the upper plate for vertical deflection, and a positive
potential should be present at the lower plate for vertical deflection. It
should be noted that the vertical and horizontal plates are independent of
one another. Therefore, the beam may be moved to any position on the
face of the CRT by using appropriate input voltages.

As mentioned above, the X axis on an oscilloscope represents time.
Therefore, if time is to be measured precisely, the sweep rate of the
electron beam in the horizontal plane must be uniform. To produce this
uniform deflection, a sawtooth waveform is applied to the horizontal
plates. The reader will recall that a sawtooth waveform increases in a linear
manner to a given point and then falls abruptly to zero amplitude. Thus,

when such a waveform is applied to the horizontal deflection plates, it causes the electron beam to move linearly from left to right across the face of the CRT. When the voltage falls to zero the electron beam moves instantaneously (with no further horizontal deflection) to its original position at the left of the screen. Since the sweep rate is uniform, the face of the CRT may be calculated in seconds/division on the graticule (faceplate) placed over the CRT. The sweep rate may be changed by adjusting the frequency (repetition rate) of the sawtooth waveform. This, of course, will alter the total time of the display on the CRT.

The vertical deflection amplifier is used to provide ample vertical gain between the input waveform and the CRT. The CRT is constructed so that it will operate properly for voltages which fall within a specified range. Therefore, the vertical deflection amplifier is preceded by an input attenuator. If the incoming signal is too high, the signal is attenuated. If, on the other hand, the signal is of low level, the input attenuation is reduced so that the signal may be amplified properly. The vertical deflection amplifier/input attenuator combination is calibrated so that a given amount of voltage will produce a specified vertical deflection on the graticule.

Several types of oscilloscopes are commonly used in the laboratory in addition to the single trace units described above. Dual trace oscilloscopes are capable of monitoring two separate waveforms simultaneously. Using these instruments, the experimenter uses the same horizontal time scale for the two waveforms, but is able to alter the input attenuation and positions of the two channels independently of one another. Storage oscilloscopes have the ability to retain a given waveform on the CRT for extended time periods. These latter instruments are particularly useful for measuring transient signals or for photographing signal displays.

Figure 2.12 shows a general purpose single trace oscilloscope (Heath IO-102).

Sound-Level Meters

Sound-level meters are essential for the measurement of sound pressure quantities (with reference to 0.0002 dyne/cm^2). These meters may be used to make sound measurements in the field or may be used in conjunction with an artificial ear to determine the sound pressures generated by an earphone.

A sound-level meter is essentially an AC voltmeter whose input voltage is generated by a microphone. That is, a typical sound-level meter consists of an omnidirectional microphone, a calibrated attenuator, an amplifier, and a moving coil meter. In addition to the flat frequency response provided by the above circuitry, several frequency weighting networks are

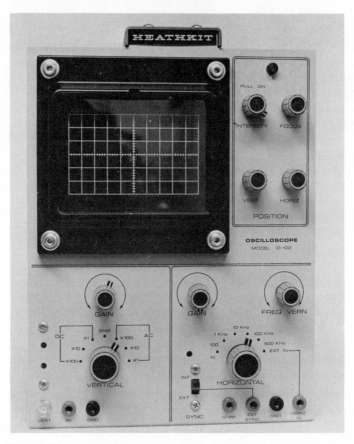

Figure 2.12. Heath IO-102 general purpose single channel oscilloscope.

also included. The purpose of these networks is to approximate the frequency response characteristics of the normal human ear. Three response curves have been internationally accepted. They are referred to as the A, B, and C frequency response curves and correspond to the inverse of the 40-, 70-, and 100-phon equal loudness contours, respectively (See Chapter 4.3). Figure 2.13 shows the A, B, and C frequency response curves. When sound pressure is measured in dB re 0.0002 dyne/cm^2 with equal weight given to all sound frequencies, the obtained readings are referred to as "X" dB *sound pressure level* (SPL). However, if a weighting network is used, the readings are referred to as "X" dB (A, B, or C) *sound level*. For example, if the A-weighting network is used, the obtained reading might be 70 dB (A). A reading of 70 dB SPL would refer to the

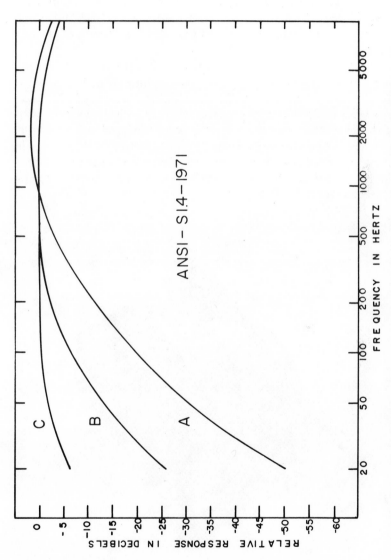

Figure 2.13. Frequency weighting response curves (American National Standards Institute (ANSI), *Sound Level Meters* S1.4-1971).

condition where a weighting network was not used. Figure 2.14*a* shows a general purpose sound-level meter (General Radio 1551-C) which may be used to make sound measurements in various sound fields. Figure 2.14*b* shows another sound-level meter (Breul and Kjaer 2203) which has been coupled to an artificial ear (Breul and Kjaer 4152) so that sound pressures generated by the earphone may be determined.

The reading from a sound-level meter tells little about the spectral composition of the sound. Some qualitative information may be gained by noting the meter response for different weighting networks. For example, if a reading on the linear scale remains relatively unchanged when measuring the same sound with the A scale, it may be inferred that most of the frequency components of the sound lie above about 1,000 Hz. Conversely, if the A-weighted reading is considerably below the linear scale value, it may be inferred that the sound contains a significant number of components below about 1,000 Hz.

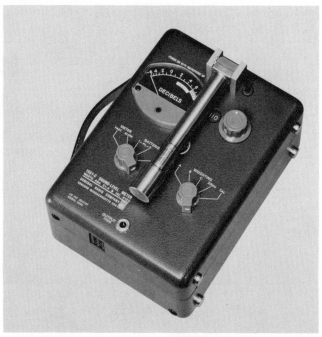

Figure 2.14*a*. General Radio 1551-C sound-level meter set up to make measurements in the sound field. Courtesy of General Radio.

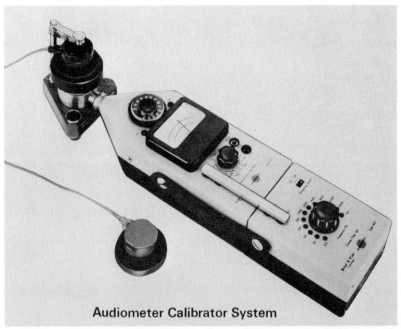

Audiometer Calibrator System

Figure 2.14*b*. Audiometer calibrator system. Breul and Kjaer 2203 attached to Breul and Kjaer 4152 artificial ear for earphone measurements. Courtesy of Breul and Kjaer.

Wave Analyzers

Wave analyzers are designed to measure the spectral composition of complex waves. This is accomplished by selectively filtering the input signal throughout the audio frequency range. The filtering process may be in the form of contiguous bands which overlap each other, or the filter may be continuously swept over the frequency range. In either case, the amplitude of the signal for each filter position is recorded (either manually or automatically) and a frequency versus amplitude plot obtained (again either manually or automatically).

Wave analyzers are classified as either constant percentage analyzers or constant bandwidth analyzers. Constant percentage analyzers are designed so that the bandwidth of the filter is always a constant proportion of the center frequency. Instruments of this variety typically incorporate one or more of the following constant percentage bandwidths: 60% (1 octave), 23% ($^1/_3$ octave), or 7% ($^1/_{10}$ octave). Constant bandwidth analyzers incorporate filter bandwidths which remain constant (in Hz) throughout the audio range. Normally, the bandwidths of these analyzers are quite narrow and may be only a few Hertz wide. For example, the General Radio model 1900-A wave analyzer has selectable bandwidths of only 3, 10, and 50 Hz.

The choice of the type of wave analyzer to be used depends upon the measurement task. Constant bandwidth analyzers are primarily intended for fine detailed analysis. For example, these instruments may be used for harmonic distortion measurements where it is necessary to isolate a single frequency component. Constant percentage analyzers are better suited for acoustic noise measurements because a finely detailed analysis is not typically required. Under these latter circumstances, an adequate noise analysis may consist simply of 1- or ⅓-octave band data.

It should be noted that the calculation of the spectrum level of a flat noise source differs somewhat using constant bandwidth and constant percentage analyzers. To determine the spectrum level using a constant bandwidth analyzer, one subtracts a constant value from the overall level of the band for all frequency regions. If, for example, the filter bandwidth is 50 Hz, the experimenter would subtract a constant value of 10.7 dB from the overall sound level (spectrum level (dB SPL/Hz) = $10 \log_{10}$ BW = $10 \log_{10} 50 = 10 \times 1.7 = 10.7$ dB). On the other hand, determination of the spectrum level using a constant percentage analyzer requires that the bandwidth of the filter for a given center frequency be determined first. Once the bandwidth is calculated, the dB value to be subtracted from the overall level may be obtained.

Figure 2.15 shows an audio frequency wave analyzer (Breul and Kjaer 2120) of the constant percentage type. The bandwidths of the analyzer may be adjusted from 1–23% of the center frequency in four steps. The input to the analyzer may be a condenser microphone or the output of a sound-level meter. Frequency analysis may be manual or automatic. In the automatic mode, a graphic level recorder is mechanically linked to the tuning dial of the analyzer. As the tuning dial is swept (by an external motor in the level recorder), the output amplitudes are automatically recorded on frequency calibrated paper. In this manner, a frequency versus amplitude plot is obtained. When used manually, the operator adjusts the tuning dial to a desired center frequency and then notes the amplitude on the built-in voltmeter. This is performed over the entire frequency range.

Graphic Level Recorders

Graphic level recorders produce permanent strip-chart records of AC voltages. In a typical graphic level recorder, different types of papers are supplied for different purposes. For recording the level of a signal over time, the paper is lined so that the ordinate is plotted linearly in decibels

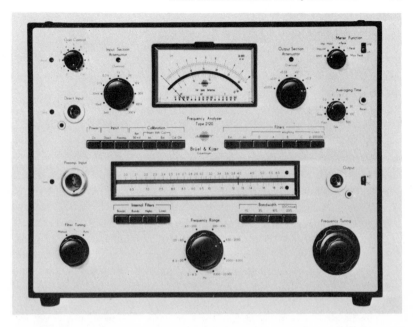

Figure 2.15. Breul and Kjaer 2120 audio frequency wave analyzer. Courtesy of Breul and Kjaer.

and the abscissa linearly lined to represent time. The speed of the paper determines the calibration along the time axis. Events which occur over long time periods would generally be recorded using slow paper speeds, while those studies which investigate transient or rapidly changing phenomena would require more rapid paper speeds. For example, in a study designed to investigate reverberation time, it is essential that the paper speed be rapid enough to separate the original sound from the reflected sound. For recording the level of a signal as a function of frequency, a second paper type is used. On these papers, the abscissa (frequency) is plotted logarithmically, while the ordinate is, once again, plotted linearly in terms of decibels. To achieve an amplitude versus frequency plot, the graphic level recorder is mechanically linked to the frequency dial of a wave analyzer (for spectral analysis) or to an oscillator (for frequency response analysis). These linkages are designed so that the frequency on the tuning dial remains synchronized with the frequency calibration on the paper as the frequency dial is swept over the entire frequency range. As the position of the frequency dial changes, so does the amplitude of the input signal to the level recorder. These amplitude changes are, of course, graphically recorded with the end-product being a complete spectral analysis. Figure 2.16 shows a laboratory-type graphic level recorder (General Radio 1521-B) which may be used in each of the modes discussed above.

Magnetic Tape Recorders

Magnetic tape recorders serve a number of useful purposes in the psychoacoustics laboratory. They may be used for both the measurement of signals as well as for the presentation of a primary signal source. When used for measurement, the original signal may be stored and then analyzed at a later time using other instruments such as an oscilloscope or wave analyzer. This is of particular importance when the acoustic event is of a transient or rapidly changing nature.

Magnetic tape recorders consist of three essential parts: the tape transport, the heads, and the electronic circuitry.

The tape transport is the mechanical part of the recorder. Its main function is to move the tape past the head assemblies at a constant and precise speed. If a constant speed is not maintained, the pitch of the sound will vary. Common tape speeds for recorders found in the laboratory and clinic are $1\frac{7}{8}$, $3\frac{3}{4}$, $7\frac{1}{2}$, and 15 inches per second.

The heads perform three functions: record, playback, and erase. Depending upon the tape recorder design, individual units may have three separate heads, one for each of the above functions, or may have two heads. In the latter case, one head serves the erase function, while the other serves both the recording and playback functions.

Magnetic tape recording and reproduction is based upon the reorientation of metallic oxide particles which are deposited on one side of a plastic

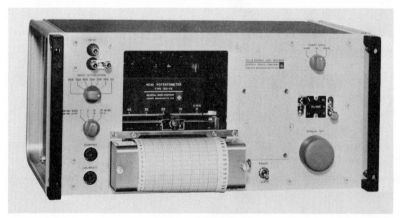

Figure 2.16. General Radio 1521-B graphic level recorder. Courtesy of General Radio.

tape. This is accomplished by the design of the heads. In general, the heads are constructed of a ring-shaped magnetic core that carries one or more coils. The core contains an air gap which is passed over by the metallic oxide coating of the moving tape. In the record condition an audio frequency current is applied to the coils. This causes corresponding alterations in the magnetic flux of the core. As the tape passes over the gap, the intensity of magnetization changes with the instantaneous amplitudes of the signal. (When recording a high frequency, bias voltage is also necessary to produce a linear response curve of the tape. This bias voltage, however, is well above the frequency limit of human hearing and is, therefore, not perceived.) In the playback (or reproduce) condition, the process is reversed; that is, as the tape passes over the air gap, a voltage is induced in the core which corresponds to the alterations in the magnetic flux of the tape. These voltage variations are then amplified to reproduce the original sound. In the erase mode, a high frequency current (about 50–100 kHz is applied to the coils, which causes the tape to return to its neutral state.

General purpose magnetic tape recorders may contain one or more amplifiers for their recording and playback functions and a high frequency bias oscillator. In an instrument which uses one head for both recording and playback, a single amplifier frequently serves both purposes; that is, when recording, the input of the amplifier is switched to accomodate the input signal so that the head may be properly energized. In the playback mode the same amplifier serves to amplify the voltages induced in the head. In recorders which have separate record and playback heads, it is usually the case that separate amplifiers are used. The bias oscillator serves two functions. The first is to supply a bias voltage during recording, while the second is to provide a high frequency current to the erase head.

Digital Counters

Digital counters have significantly improved the precision and convenience of making both frequency and time interval measurements in the laboratory. The numerical readouts from these instruments provide a clear and unambiguous display ordinarily not obtained using conventional analog instrumentation.

Counters consist of a number of functional parts, each with a specific purpose. These include decade counting units (DCUs), the time base or clock, the main gate, and the decade divider assemblies. The *decade counting units* serve to totalize the number of input pulses in a given time period and to present this total in the form of a numerical display. These displays may take the form of an in-line arrangement of gas-filled Nixie tubes or light-emitting diode (LED) displays among others. The *time base* or *clock* is typically a quartz crystal oscillator which serves as a reference standard of time. The *main gate* controls the time period during which the DCUs may totalize the input pulses. Finally, the decade divider assemblies (DCAs) control the gate time.

Frequency measurements are obtained by first converting each cycle of the input frequency to a sharp pulse using a Schmitt signal shaper. The main gate is then opened for a precise time period. This period is typically 1 second for audio frequency work. During the time the gate is open, the number of pulses is totalized and numerically displayed. Thus, if the input frequency is 1,000 Hz, the Schmitt trigger arrangement will produce 1,000 input pulses during the 1-second interval that the gate is open.

Time interval measurements are obtained by having the unknown input signal control the main gate time, while the time base frequency is counted using the DCUs. This, of course, is accomplished by reversing the input and time base connections. The resulting display may be read in seconds, milliseconds, or microseconds depending upon the period and frequency of the time base generator.

Figure 2.17 shows a photograph of a counter (General Radio 1192-B)

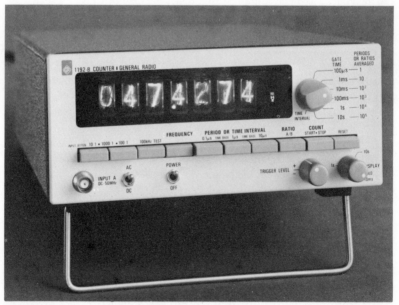

Figure 2.17. General Radio 1192-B digital frequency counter. Courtesy of General Radio.

which displays both frequency and time measurements in the manner discussed above.

REFERENCES

Beraneck, L. L. 1949. Acoustic Measurements. John Wiley & Sons, New York.

Cooke, N.E. 1960. Basic Mathematics for Electronics. McGraw-Hill, New York. 697 p.

Crowhurst, N. H. 1958. Audio Measurements. Gernsback Library, New York. 224 p.

Hewlett-Packard. 1968. Acoustics Handbook. Hewlett-Packard Company, Palo Alto, California. 118 p.

Lenk, J. D. 1969. Handbook of Practical Electronic Tests and Measurements. Prentice-Hall, Engelwood Cliffs, N. J. 302 p.

Malmstadt, H. V., C. G. Enke, and E. C. Toren, Jr. 1963. Electronics for Scientists. W. A. Benjamin, New York. 619 p.

Orr, W. I. 1967. Radio Handbook. 17th Ed. Editors and Engineers. New Augusta, Indiana. 847 p.

Peterson, A. P. G., and E. E. Gross. 1972. Handbook of Noise Measurement. 7th Ed. General Radio Co., Concord, Mass. 332 p.

Prensky, S. D. 1971. Electronic Instrumentation. 2nd Ed. Prentice-Hall, Engelwood Cliffs, N. J. 536 p.

Sarbacher, R. 1959. Encyclopedic Dictionary of Electronic and Nuclear Engineering. Prentice-Hall, Engelwood Cliffs, N. J.

chapter 3

BLOCK DIAGRAMMING OF EXPERIMENTAL APPARATUS

The arrangement of the apparatus in a psychoacoustic investigation follows a sequence that is primarily based upon the objective of the study. That is, the purpose of the study will dictate: 1) the primary signal source to be used, 2) the type of signal shaping to be used, 3) the type of transducer to be used, and 4) how the results are to be measured. With the above clearly in mind, the experimenter may block out the equipment arrangement. Block diagramming simply entails the use of symbols and lines to represent the input and output connections among the various circuit components. Blocking in this manner is useful in assuring that, when the actual interconnections are made, they will be made in the most effective and logical manner possible. Figure 3.1 shows the block diagram symbols that will be used throughout this text. It should be noted that the connecting wires between the various components should be shielded to avoid the introduction of spurious electrical signals. Furthermore, each of the components should be connected to a common ground point. This may be accomplished by attending to the positive and negative terminals at the inputs and outputs of most laboratory instruments. When binding posts are used as the input or output terminals, the positive side is frequently color-coded red while the grounded (negative) side is colored black. If color coding is not used, the symbol ($\perp$) indicates the ground side.

Perhaps the simplest apparatus arrangement used in psychoacoustics is used in the determination of absolute threshold for pure tones. In this case, the apparatus may be blocked, as seen in Figure 3.2.

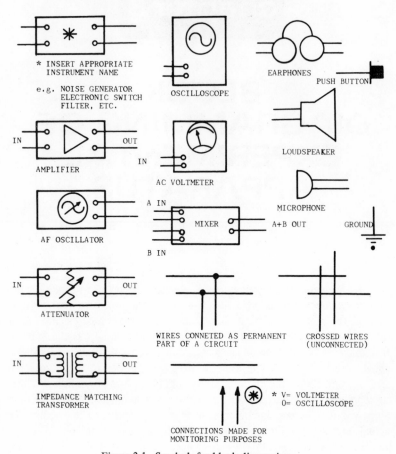

Figure 3.1. Symbols for block diagraming.

Figure 3.2 shows the oscillator to be the signal source. It is assumed that the oscillator output is not of sufficient magnitude to drive the transducer to a desired level. Therefore, an amplifier is introduced directly after the oscillator. Following the amplifier is an attenuator which is capable of attenuating voltage in dB steps. The attenuator output is led directly to the subject's earphone. (The reader is advised that for simplicity of presentation it is assumed that the various input and output impedances of the circuit components are matched. In practice, however, it is often the case that an impedance mismatch will occur. For example, in Figure 3.2, the attenuator might have an output impedance of 600 ohms, while the earphone impedance may be only 10 ohms. An impedance-

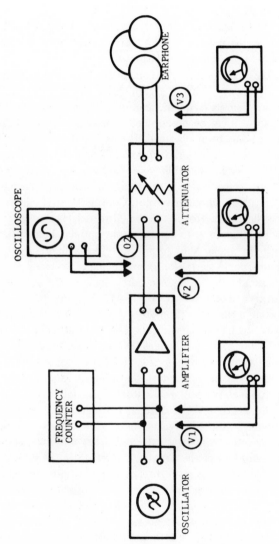

Figure3.2.   Absolute thresholds for pure tones (block diagram).

matching transformer would then be inserted between these two devices to correct the mismatch.) The subject may be seated in an adjacent room or in close proximity to the experimenter. Quiet conditions must, of course, be maintained at all times.

Auditory thresholds are commonly determined in dB SPL. The following describes how the present apparatus arrangement may be calibrated so that the threshold level is read in dB SPL.

The first step in calibrating the apparatus is to set the oscillator to the desired audio frequency. This is accomplished simply by monitoring the output frequency using a frequency counter. If a frequency counter is not available, frequency may be determined using an oscilloscope. After the desired frequency has been obtained, the oscillator voltage is raised to a level which adequately drives the amplifier. Recall that the output of an untuned amplifier should faithfully reproduce the input waveform. If the input signal from the oscillator is too weak, an inadequate signal-to-noise ratio will occur at the amplifier output. Conversely, if the input signal is too high, the signal waveform will be distorted (peak-clipped) at the amplifier output. Therefore, to determine the optimal input voltage to the amplifier, both the input and output waveforms should be monitored using an oscilloscope. Once the optimum oscillator voltage level has been determined, it should remain unchanged throughout the remainder of the experiment (i.e., V_1 should remain constant).

The next step in the calibration process is to set the attenuator to 0-dB attenuation and then to place the earphone in an artificial ear (NBS 9-A coupler). At this point the gain (intensity) control on the amplifier may be adjusted so that a predetermined SPL at the earphone is obtained. For example, the experimenter may adjust the amplifier gain to produce 80 dB SPL at the earphone. The voltage at point V_2 is noted. This voltage will equal that found at point V_3 because no attenuation is present. Assuming that the attenuator is correctly calibrated (that is, will introduce the amount of attenuation shown on the dial face), the experimenter may remove the earphone from the coupler. To determine the subject's threshold, either the subject or experimenter (depending upon the experimental design) turns the attenuator until the audible threshold is reached. The threshold level in dB SPL is simply the original SPL value with no attenuation present minus the new attenuation value. For example, 0.5 volt at point V_2 may yield 80 dB SPL for a 1,000-Hz tone with no attenuation in the circuit. If 72-dB additional attenuation is required to reach the threshold for a given subject, the threshold level is 8 dB SPL. In order for the apparatus to remain in calibration, the voltage at point V_2 must remain constant.

A somewhat more complex arrangement of the experimental apparatus used to measure auditory thresholds may be seen in Figure 3.3. This design is capable of presenting pulsed (interrupted) tones rather than continuous tones as in Figure 3.2. Thus, adaptation effects, which might have influenced the results using the previous design, are reduced using the present arrangement.

Before continuing with the present circuit, it is worthwhile to backtrack for a moment and consider why the tones in the previous circuit (Figure 3.2) could not be interrupted by a simple switch placed just before the subject's headphone. The answer, of course, is that such a switch would introduce spurious transients at the initiation and termination of each tone presentation because of the extremely rapid rise and fall times. The reader will recall that such transients have energy contents which extend well above and below the frequency of interest. It is, therefore, a strong possibility that, if such an arrangement were used, the subject might respond to the click-like transient rather than to the tone. This, of course, would bias the results.

Figure 3.3 shows the audio oscillator output being fed to the input of the electronic switch. The electronic switch interrupts the stimulus at a chosen rate and controls the rise and fall times. It is assumed that the electronic switch output is not of sufficient magnitude to adequately drive the transducer. Therefore, an amplifier follows the electronic switch. (If the electronic switch output could sufficiently drive the transducer to a high enough output level, the amplifier could be removed from the circuit.) In the present design, two attenuators are included, one in the experimenter's control room and the other in the subject's test room. The use of two attenuators allows for more variation of the experimental conditions, as will be discussed below. After being directed through both attenuators (whose attenuation settings combine), the signal is routed to a single earphone.

Calibration using the present design is similar to that used in the previous design. A voltage capable of driving the electronic switch is adjusted using the gain control on the oscillator. This voltage (V_1) must remain constant throughout the experiment. The output voltage from the electronic switch is then set to a level capable of driving the amplifier. This voltage (V_2) should also remain constant. (For calibration purposes, the electronic switch may be set to a "constant on" position.) Furthermore, the signal waveform at the electronic switch output (O_1) should be monitored. At this point the earphone may be mounted in an artificial ear assembly, and both attenuators set to 0-dB attenuation. The gain control on the amplifier is then rotated until a predetermined SPL is obtained. The

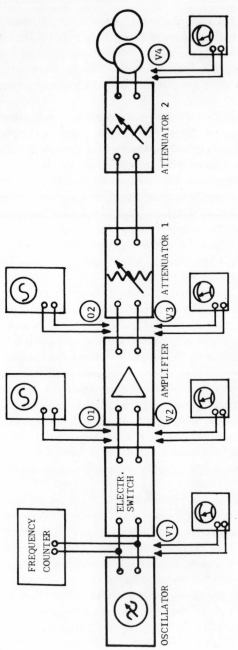

Figure 3.3. Apparatus for pure tone thresholds (interrupted tones).

voltage producing this SPL is noted (V_3) and should remain constant. With no attenuation in the circuit, the voltage just before the earphone (V_4) should equal V_3. The amplifier output is checked for distortion using an oscilloscope (O_2). Assuming that both attenuators are linear, any threshold level may now be determined simply by subtracting the attenuation settings from the initial SPL reading with no attenuation in the circuit.

When threshold is determined using a method in which the subject controls the stimulus level (to be fully discussed in Chapter 4), it is desirable to change the relative position of the subject's dial setting from trial to trial. This is because the subject may gain positional cues which might bias the experimental results. To reduce this bias the experimenter may change the attenuation setting of attenuator 1 from time to time. To illustrate, the experimenter may first introduce 30-dB attenuation using attenuator 1 and have the subject adjust attenuator 2 to his audible threshold. The combined settings of attenuators 1 and 2 would then be subtracted from the original SPL value to determine the threshold level. After several threshold determinations, it is possible that the subject will use the relative position of his previous dial settings in making further judgments. The subject may be aware or unaware of this bias. In any event, the bias is reduced by changing the attenuation value of attenuator 1. Since the threshold dB SPL is the original SPL minus the combined attenuation, the position of the subject's attenuator knob will change, but the total attenuation will not. (To further reduce response bias, the numerical values printed on the attenuator face plate used by the subject should be obscured. In addition, the subject's attenuator should be continuously variable with no detents.)

The apparatus arrangements which have been presented to this point are used for the determination of the absolute threshold for pure tones in quiet. In psychoacoustic research, however, it is frequently the case that noise is introduced together with the pure tones. The purpose of these studies is frequently to determine the relation between the noise (i.e., masker) level and the pure tone threshold. The noises used most often in these studies are either white-noise or narrow-band noise. Figure 3.4 shows a block diagram of the equipment used to determine the effects of narrow-band noise on the pure tone threshold. (The block diagram symbols for both voltmeters and oscilloscopes have been replaced at several points in the figure to avoid cluttering. These measurement points, however, are noted by either a circled "V" (voltmeter) or "O" (oscilloscope) together with a number. This practice will be followed throughout the remainder of the text.)

The apparatus may be divided into two circuits whose outputs are

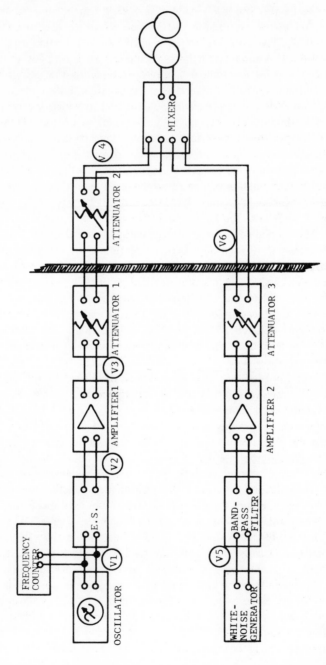

Figure 3.4. Apparatus to determine pure tone thresholds in noise.

mixed just before the earphone. The tone circuit is identical to that used in Figure 3.3. The noise circuit consists of a white-noise generator, a filter in the band-pass mode, an amplifier, and an attenuator. The output from the attenuator is then mixed with the output of the tone circuit. It is decided that the limiting frequencies of the noise will be 600 and 1,200 Hz. The test frequency is 1,000 Hz.

Calibration of the tone circuit is identical to that discussed for the previous figure. However, during calibration of the tone circuit, attenuator 3 should be at its maximum attenuation setting to prevent the noise from interfering. Calibration of the noise circuit is accomplished in a similar fashion as the tone circuit. An adequate voltage from the noise generator is applied to the input of the amplifier (V_5). With attenuator 3 set to 0-dB attenuation, the gain on the amplifier is increased so that a predetermined sound level is produced by the earphone. The voltage at point V_6 is noted and should remain the same whenever attenuator 3 is in the 0-dB attenuation position. (The voltage at V_6 will, of course, decrease as attenuator 3 is varied.) During calibration of the noise circuit, attenuators 1 and 2 should be set to maximum attenuation to prevent the pure tone stimuli from interfering with the noise SPL readings.

It has been mentioned at several points during this chapter that it is extremely important for attenuators to be calibrated, i.e., to attenuate signals by the amount indicated on the attenuator dial plate. The following paragraph introduces the reader to basic attenuator calibration procedures.

The process by which an attenuator in a circuit may be calibrated is relatively simple and may be accomplished using either voltage or SPL measures. When using voltage measurements, an arbitrary voltage is applied to the system from the signal source. The attenuator is then set to 0-dB attenuation. For example, 1 volt from the amplifier output in Figure 3.2 may be applied to the remainder of the circuit (V_2 = 1 volt). With the attenuator set to 0 dB, V_3 will also be 1 volt. Attenuation is then introduced in 10-dB steps. If the attenuator is in calibration, its output voltage should drop 10 dB (to about 0.3 volt). With an additional 10-dB attenuation, the voltage at V_3 should drop to 0.1 volt. This process is continued until the entire attenuation range is traversed. To calculate the correct voltage for any attenuator setting, the equation:

$$N_{dB} = 20 \log \frac{V_1}{V_2}$$

may be used, where V_1 is the original voltage and V_2 is the obtained voltage at the attenuator output (Peterson, A. P. G., and E. E. Gross, 1972. Handbook of Noise Measurement, pp. 248–9. General Radio Concord).

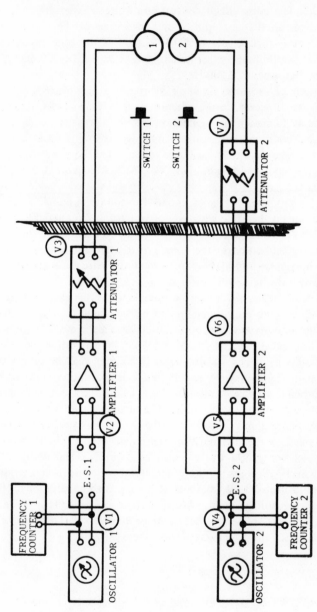

Figure 3.5. Block diagram for equipment used to obtain binaural loudness balances with two oscillators.

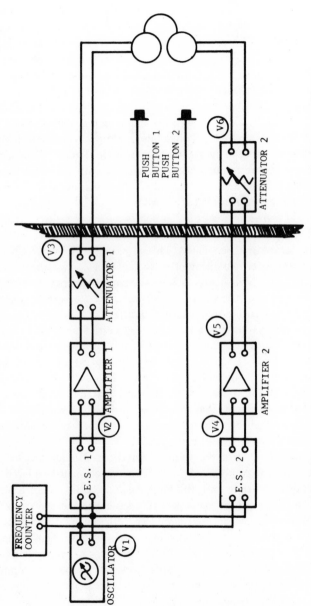

Figure 3.6. Block diagram for equipment used to obtain binaural loudness balances with one oscillator.

obtained readings are different from the calculated values, the difference (in dB) is taken into account in the calibration. A simpler method for calibrating an attenuator is simply to read the SPL output for various attenuator settings. For example, the same 1 volt reference voltage at point V_2 in Figure 3.2 may produce 100 dB SPL at the earphone with 0-dB attenuation present. When attenuation is introduced, the SPL at the earphone should be reduced in an equivalent amount. If not, the actual dB values are noted.

To this point, each of the three experimental circuits have been designed to investigate monaural phenomena. Many experiments, however, explore relations between two ears. For example, loudness balances between two sounds are frequently investigated in both the laboratory and clinic. Figures 3.5 and 3.6 show two block diagrams which can be used to investigate loudness balances between two ears.

The circuit shown in Figure 3.5 is somewhat more versatile than that shown in Figure 3.6 in that the frequencies of the tones delivered to each ear may be varied independently. This is particularly useful when balancing the loudness of two different frequency tones, as when determining isophonic contours (see Chapter 4.3). If the same frequency is to be heard in both ears, however, the circuit shown in Figure 3.6 is preferable since there is no chance that the frequencies will differ.

The equipment arrangements in both Figures 3.5 and 3.6 are uncomplicated. In the first arrangement, two oscillators feed separate channels of an electronic switch. Each channel may be turned on or off by an individual lever switch in the subject's room. The durations of the tones are controlled by the subject. (It is assumed that the electronic switch includes two independent channels, each of which is capable of being externally controlled by the subject. In this mode of operation, the purpose of the switch is merely to control the rise and fall times of the tones, but not to control the stimulus durations. If such an electronic switch is not available, a conventional lever switch may be placed after each oscillator in order to turn the tones on and off. To reduce transients introduced by the switches, band-pass filters (centered at the frequencies being used) should precede each amplifier in the circuit.) The electronic switch outputs are then led to individual amplifiers and then to separate attenuators. The reader should note that attenuator 1 is controlled by the experimenter and attenuator 2 by the subject. The attenuator outputs are then led to their respective earphones. The subject's task is to balance the loudness of a comparison tone (represented by the lower half of the circuit) to the loudness of a standard tone (represented by the upper half of the circuit). The only difference between Figures 3.5 and 3.6 is that in the latter design the oscillator output is split and utilized in both channels.

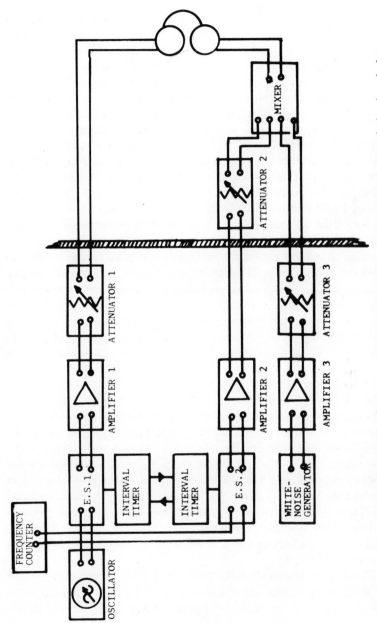

Figure 3.7. Block diagram for equipment used to obtain binaural loudness balance between unmasked and masked tone.

Calibration of the apparatus in Figures 3.5 and 3.6 in terms of sound pressure level is identical to that presented for Figures 3.3 and 3.4. However, if calibration is to be in terms of dB SL (sensation level), a somewhat different procedure is used. The procedure is initiated by first setting the electronic switch so that the tone pulses alternate at a rate of about 500 msec on and 500 msec off (25 msec rise- and fall-times). Each channel is calibrated individually by first adjusting the attenuator to the subject's threshold. For example, if channel 1 (standard channel) in Figure 3.6 were to be calibrated in dB SL, the experimenter might use an "Up-Down" procedure (see Chapter 4.1) to obtain the subject's threshold. The attenuator setting associated with the threshold level would then be noted. If the attenuation were then to be reduced by "X" dB, the SL of the signal would equal that number. Thus, if the attenuation were reduced 35 dB, the SL would also be 35 dB. It should be remembered that, during the calibration of one channel, the attenuator in the opposite channel should be set to maximum to avoid interference.

In another type of loudness balancing experiment, a tone is balanced in loudness with a second tone which is presented in a noise background. The purpose of this type of experiment is to ascertain how loudness grows in masked ears as compared with loudness growth in unmasked ears. The results of such experiments have both theoretical and practical implications concerning hearing in normal and pathological listeners. Figure 3.7 shows a block diagram of the equipment used in such a loudness-balancing experiment.

A tone alone (channel 1) is automatically alternated with a tone-in-noise (channel 2). The durations and rise- and fall-times of the tones in both channels are identical. The electronic switches are controlled by separate interval timers which are wired together so that they trigger each other. Unlike the two previous designs, the subjects cannot control the presentation times of the tones. To illustrate, an unmasked (standard) tone may be presented for 2 seconds to one ear, followed 500 msec later by a 2-second masked tone presented to the opposite ear. The subject's task is to balance the loudness of the masked tone (using attenuator 2) to the loudness of the unmasked tone. Note that in the present design the noise remains on constantly in the masked ear. Only the tones will alternate between ears.

The circuits presented in the present chapter represent only a few of the many arrangements which may be used in psychoacoustic and audiological research. If the reader has become familiar with the basic designs presented here, he will be well on his way to understanding more complex arrangements.

chapter 4

CLASSICAL AREAS IN PSYCHOACOUSTICS WITH REPRESENTATIVE EXPERIMENTS

The primary objective of this chapter is to demonstrate how a psycho-acoustic experiment is designed and conducted. The format is first to acquaint the reader with a classical subject area, with emphasis placed upon the methodologies used to investigate the area. The introductory material is followed by a detailed description of an experiment in the area. The primary intent of these illustrative experiments is to provide the student with models which he or she can use in performing similar experiments. Typically, each experiment includes step-by-step descriptions of: 1) the equipment arrangement, 2) calibration procedures, 3) methodological procedures, and 4) data analaysis.

4.1. ABSOLUTE THRESHOLD MEASUREMENT

A common problem in psychoacoustics is to determine the lowest stimulus value that an observer can perceive, i.e., the absolute threshold. The classical view of the absolute threshold (often abbreviated RL from the German *Reiz Limen*) is that of an all-or-none phenomenon. That is, a critical level of neural activity must be surpassed at the brain center associated with a given receptor organ for a stimulus to be perceived. If a stimulus falling on a receptor does not produce the critical central effect, it will not be perceived. The early psychophysicists were among the first to realize, however, that the absolute threshold was not only subject to much variation among individuals, but was also subject to considerable variation within a given individual. Variability within a subject is governed by a multitude of internal (intrinsic) and external (extrinsic) factors which, theoretically, vary randomly from trial to trial, thereby altering the critical level. This, in turn, will cause the obtained behavioral threshold to be distributed in a more-or-less statistically normal manner about a central stimulus value. Because of this inherent variability, the measurement of absolute thresholds may best be defined statistically as the mean of repeated measures. Thus, an operational definition of the absolute threshold is the minimum stimulus value which will elicit a response half (50%) of the time. Table 4.1 lists various intrinsic and extrinsic factors which may govern momentary variations in auditory threshold sensitivity.

Classical Procedures

Three psychophysical methods have been extensively used in determining both absolute and differential thresholds. Although the methods differ, each is designed to obtain repeated thresholds and to extract an overall mean value.

The Method of Limits (or the Method of Minimal Changes) is based upon ascending and descending stimulus series. The stimuli about the assumed threshold are either increased or decreased in equal increments.

Table 4.1. Some factors that cause momentary variations in auditory thresholds

Factors	Variations
"Physiological noise"	Pulse noises, vascular noises, breathing, tinnitus (head noises) may change from moment to moment
Motivation	The motivation to perform the task may change from moment to moment
Attention	Attention may vary from moment to moment
Signal criterion	Different qualities of the signal may be responded to on different trials
Practice	The threshold may improve as a function of practice
Environmental changes	The environment in which the test is being done may change, thereby influencing the measured threshold
Methodology	A difference between ascending and descending trials affects the threshold level

The subject's task is simply to report whether or not the stimulus is perceived. Generally, six or more stimulus series are included. Table 4.2 shows the use of the Method of Limits in determining the threshold for one individual using 250-Hz tones.

The results obtained in the experiment are measured in six stimulus series, three ascending and three descending. The stimuli are presented in 2-dB SPL steps and range from 2–28 dB SPL. In such an experiment the experimenter must know beforehand the probable stimulus values for threshold. This may be accomplished by pretesting several subjects or by referring to values determined in other investigations. Table 4.2 shows that the experimenter first used an ascending stimulus series. In such a series the level of the stimuli are initially below the subject's assumed threshold. The first stimulus in this series was 10 dB SPL which did not produce a response. Thus, a negative sign (−) is placed in the appropriate position in the table. The next stimulus (12 dB SPL) was then presented. This stimulus value did not produce a response, and another negative sign is indicated. The series was continued until 20 dB SPL was reached, at which

Table 4.2. Threshold measurement using the Method of Limits for one individual (250-Hz tones)

Stimulus value in dB SPL	Stimulus series					
	Asc.[a]	Des.	Asc.	Des.	Asc.	Des.
28	+	+				+
26	+	+				+
24	+	+	+		+	+
22	+	+	+	+	+	+
20	+	+	+	+	−	+
18	−	+	+	+	−	+
16	−	−	−	−	−	−
14	−	−	−	−	−	−
12	−	−	−	−		−
10	−	−		−		−
8		−		−		−
6		−				
4		−				
2		−				
Series threshold[b]	19.0	17.0	17.0	17.0	21.0	19.0

[a]Asc., ascending; des., descending.
[b]Overall mean threshold = 18.3 dB SPL; standard deviation = 1.7 dB.

time the subject indicated that a tone was heard. At this point a positive sign (+) is indicated. The series was continued to 28 dB SPL with all values yielding positive responses. The first descending series was then initiated above the assumed threshold level and continued until the stimulus level was well below threshold. In this particular descending series, the stimuli were presented at all values from 28 dB to 2 dB SPL (the series end-points). It should be noted, however, that neither the first nor last stimulus to be presented in an ascending or descending series does not necessarily have to be the end-point for that series. In fact, the series should be adjusted to avoid various biases which this method would introduce had the series end-points always been the same.

The Method of Limits is particularly sensitive to two biasing factors which may lead to consistent over- or underestimations of the absolute threshold. The first factor (or *constant error*) is the *error of habituation*. If the error of habituation is present, the subject may fall into the "habit" of continuing to respond "no" in an ascending stimulus series and "yes" in a descending stimulus series. This, of course, would lead to a higher threshold level in the former instance and a lower threshold level in the latter instance. The second constant error which may occur is the *error of anticipation*. If such an error is present, the subject would tend to respond prematurely simply because he or she expects a change to occur. For example, in an ascending series, the subject may report "yes" simply because he has anticipated it. In fact, the level of the stimulus may still be below threshold. Conversely, in a descending series, the subject may prematurely report "no" simply on the basis of expectation. The errors of anticipation and habituation may be minimized by using a relatively large number of ascending and descending series in order to average out these probable constant errors. The errors may be minimized further by varying the end-points of the stimulus series.

The absolute threshold for each stimulus series is determined by calculating the series transition (T) point. The T point is the midpoint between the last negative (−) response and the first positive (+) response in the series. Thus, for the first ascending series in Table 4.2, the first positive response was 20 dB SPL and the last negative response was 18 dB SPL. The series threshold was then 19 dB SPL. To determine an overall threshold for the six series, all six T values are averaged. The overall threshold for this subject was 18.33 dB SPL for the 250-Hz tones. The standard deviation of the obtained T values may be used as a measure of the variability of the threshold responses. For this example, the standard deviation was 1.73 dB.

The Method of Constant Stimuli differs from the Method of Limits in that ascending and descending series are not included. Instead, about five to eight stimuli are chosen which lie above and below the assumed threshold. The method further requires that the distance between each of the stimuli be equal. The stimuli, rather than being presented in a set series, are presented in a random order. Each stimulus is presented an equal number of times. Table 4.3 shows how the Method of Constant Stimuli may be used to determine the absolute threshold for one individual. The stimuli in this case are 4,000-Hz tones.

In the example, seven stimulus values are chosen and 20 trials per stimulus value are recorded. A positive (+) sign indicates that the subject perceived the tone and a negative (−) sign indicates that the tone was inaudible. It should be emphasized that the tones are presented in a

Table 4.3. Threshold measurement using the Method of Constant Stimuli for one individual (4,000-Hz tones)

Trial number	Stimulus value in dB SPL						
	4	6	8	10	12	14	16
1	−	−	+	+	+	−	+
2	−	−	−	+	+	+	+
3	−	−	−	−	+	+	+
4	−	−	+	+	+	−	+
5	−	−	+	−	−	+	+
6	−	−	−	−	+	+	+
7	−	+	−	+	+	+	+
8	−	−	−	−	+	+	+
9	−	+	+	−	+	−	+
10	−	−	+	−	+	+	+
11	−	+	−	+	−	+	+
12	−	−	−	−	−	+	+
13	−	−	−	−	−	+	+
14	−	−	+	+	−	+	+
15	−	−	−	+	+	+	+
16	−	−	−	−	−	+	+
17	−	−	−	+	+	+	+
18	−	−	−	−	+	+	+
19	−	−	−	+	−	−	+
20	−	−	−	−	+	+	+
Percent (+)	0	15	30	45	65	80	100

random order and not in a series. Thus, the 14-dB SPL tone may be presented first, followed by a 6-dB SPL tone, and so on until the entire 7 X 20 matrix is filled. Threshold calculation is initiated by noting the percentage of positive responses for each constant stimulus value. Once these values have been calculated, a psychometric function is plotted which relates the percentage of positive responses (on the ordinate) to the stimulus value (on the abscissa). Figure 4.1 shows the data collected in Table 4.3. Since the absolute threshold is operationally defined as that stimulus value which elicits a response half the time, a line is projected from the 50% point on the ordinate to the plotted function and then vertically to the abscissa. The point at which the vertical line intercepts the abscissa is taken as the absolute threshold. In Figure 4.1 the absolute threshold is 10.5 dB SPL.

The Method of Average Error (or the Method of Adjustment) is the least complex of the classical methods used to determine threshold. Whereas both the Methods of Limits and Constant Stimuli require that the experimenter control the stimulus levels presented to the subject, the Method of Average Error allows the subject direct control of the intensity

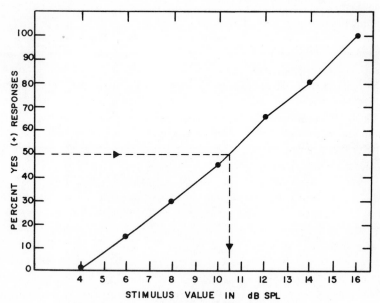

Figure 4.1. Psychometric function relating percentage of "yes" responses to stimulus intensity (in dB SPL) using the Method of Constant Stimuli.

levels. For example, when determining the absolute threshold, the subject is provided with a variable attenuator to adjust the stimulus level.

The Method of Average Error requires both ascending and descending trials. On an ascending trial the subject adjusts the stimulus intensity to audibility from an initially inaudible level. On a descending trial the stimulus is, at first, clearly audible, but is then adjusted by the subject to inaudibility. The point at which the stimulus becomes audible in an ascending trial, or inaudible in a descending trial, is taken as the threshold level for the trial. The purpose for including both ascending and descending trials is to average out subject response biases which are associated with both trial types. For example, in descending trials, subjects frequently adjust the stimulus level to lower values than on ascending trials. This is similar to the problem of habituation encountered using the Method of Limits.

Table 4.4 shows the results of a threshold determination experiment for one subject using 500-Hz tone bursts. As indicated in the table, the subject made 20 threshold judgments. Half of the trials were ascending and the other half were descending. The mean of the 20 trials was 9.75 dB SPL. This value is taken as the absolute threshold for the 500-Hz tones. The standard deviation of the obtained threshold values may be taken as a measure of the variability of the threshold judgments. The calculated value in this instance was 1.41 dB.

Variants of the Classical Procedures

One of the conditions necessary for use of either the Method of Limits or the Method of Constant Stimuli is some notion of the area in which the threshold lies. Thus, an experiment using these procedures consists, in effect, of two separate experiments. The first determines the general stimulus value for threshold, while the second determines the threshold itself. To eliminate the need for pretesting, several variants of the classical procedures have been developed.

The *Staircase Method* (or *Up-Down* procedure) is a variant of the Method of Limits. In this method the subject is instructed to make one of two judgments, "Yes, I perceive the signal" or "No, I don't perceive the signal." Threshold determination is initiated by the experimenter presenting a stimulus which he feels is close to the threshold level. The subject then reports whether the signal was perceived or not. If the stimulus is not perceived, the experimenter increases the stimulus level by a predetermined step size (e.g., 1 dB). The subject then makes another judgment. If the stimulus is not perceived, the stimulus level is increased another step. This continues until the subject reports that the signal was perceived. At

Table 4.4. Threshold measurement using the Method of Average Error for one individual (500-Hz tones)[a]

Trial number	Trial mode	Threshold in dB SPL
1	A	11
2	D	10
3	A	12
4	D	10
5	A	10
6	D	8
7	A	9
8	D	8
9	A	10
10	D	10
11	A	13
12	D	12
13	A	10
14	D	9
15	A	9
16	D	9
17	A	8
18	D	8
19	A	10
20	D	9

[a]Mean threshold = 9.75 dB SPL; standard deviation = 1.41 dB.

this time, the stimulus level is reduced one step and another judgment is made. Thus, the Staircase Method dictates that the stimulus level presented on one trial be governed by the response on the previous trial. Whenever the threshold is crossed (i.e., a change from a "Yes" to a "No," or vice versa) the direction of the stimulus step is changed. The Staircase Method is continued over a predetermined number of trials, each trial representing a step change and a judgment. The threshold is the mean of the presented stimuli. Figure 4.2 presents the results for one individual. The calculated mean threshold is 8.90 dB SPL for the 2,000-Hz tone bursts.

A variation of the Staircase Method is the threshold tracking procedure as used with a Bekesy audiometer. In this method, the subject is provided with a switch which controls a motor-driven attenuator. The attenuator is mechanically coupled to a pen which records the attenuator settings at each moment. Whenever the switch is pressed, the signal level is attenuated

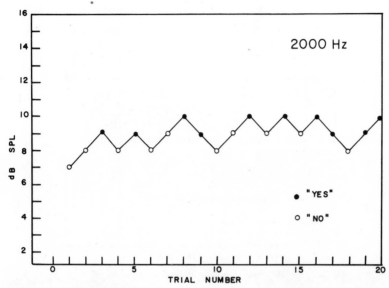

Figure 4.2. Results of a threshold measurement experiment using the Staircase Method.

(reduced) at a given rate (e.g., 2 dB/second). Conversely, when the switch is released, the attenuation is reduced (intensity increased) at the same rate. The subject's task is to track his threshold by holding the switch down wever the tone (either pulsed or on continuously) is audible and to release the switch whenever the tone is inaudible. Figure 4.3 shows the results of a hypothetical threshold determination using the tracking method. Note that the record has a sawtooth appearance. The peaks of the tracings which are closest to the lower attenuation values (greater intensities) represent the transition from inaudibility to audibility, while those peaks which are closest to the higher attenuation settings (lower intensities) represent the transition from audibility to inaudibility. The overall threshold value may be calculated by averaging the values associated with the peak points, or a median value may be obtained by drawing a line through the midpoint of the excursions.

Absolute Threshold for Pure Tones

The effective stimulus for the sense of hearing is, of course, pressure changes. Thus, the principal problem in the measurement of auditory intensive sensitivity is to determine the least SPL which will be heard 50% of the time by the subject. However, the SPL which is just capable of

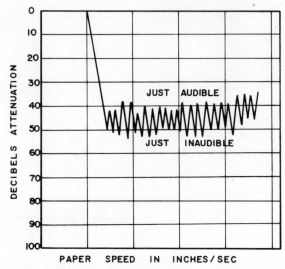

Figure 4.3. Tracking Method illustration.

eliciting sensation may be measured differently, depending upon the transducer used to generate the acoustic signals.

The *minimal audible field* (MAF) condition is generally used when loudspeakers are used to generate the sounds. In this particular procedure the subject is placed in a free sound field and oriented at a fixed angle toward the sound source. Testing for pure tones is done one frequency at a time. Any one of the previously discussed psychophysical methods may be used to determine the absolute threshold. For example, the Staircase Method might be used. In this case, the level of the stimuli would vary as dictated by the subject's responses. The mean attenuation setting corresponding to the threshold level would then be calculated and set by the experimenter. Following this, the subject is removed from the sound field. The SPL corresponding to the threshold level is then measured by inserting a calibrated microphone at the point in space previously occupied by the center of the subject's head.

The *minimal audible pressure* (MAP) condition is used when earphones are used as the transducers. The primary objective of this method is to determine the least sound pressure level at or near the tympanic membrane which is capable of eliciting a response. As in the MAF condition, any appropriate psychophysical measurement procedure may be used to determine the threshold. Once the threshold determination has been made, the experimenter may remove the earphone from the subject's head and couple it to an artificial ear (NBS 9-A coupler). The artificial ear is designed to present to the earphone an acoustic impedance which is equivalent to the average human ear. Therefore, the sound pressures generated within the coupler will approximate those which would have been obtained had a probe microphone been placed into the entrance of the ear canal under the earphone. Figure 4.4 shows the MAP reference threshold levels published by the American National Standards Institute (ANSI) in 1969. These data represent the mean threshold levels (in dB SPL) for a large group of otologically normal young adults at sound frequencies between 125 and 8,000 Hz. The values plotted in Figure 4.4 represent the SPLs produced when a Telephonics TDH-39 earphone is mounted in an MX-41/AR cushion and then coupled to a standard NBS 9-A coupler. This earphone and cushion combination is used often in both the auditory clinic and in the laboratory. The ANSI standard also specifies the reference levels for other commonly used earphones such as the Permoflux PDR-8, PDR-10, and the Western Electric 705-A.

The determination of absolute thresholds at frequencies above 8,000 Hz presents difficulties not encountered at the lower frequencies. The first problem relates to the inability of commonly used earphones in the clinic and laboratory to generate sufficiently high enough sound pressures at high frequencies. In general, a clinical type earphone (such as the TDH-39) will only have a bandwidth of about 6,000 Hz. The second problem encountered at the higher frequencies relates to standing wave patterns which may be produced when earphones are placed over the ear canals. Recently, however, relatively reliable transducers have been developed which permit high frequency thresholds to be measured (Harris and Myers, 1971). These MAP thresholds have been found to agree closely with MAF threshold levels (the preferred method for testing high frequency sensitivity before reliable MAP measures).

Corso (1965) determined the high frequency thresholds of 72 normal hearing young adults. The MAF technique was employed. Thresholds were determined for the right ear at nine test frequencies between 6,000 and 23,000 Hz. Figure 4.5 shows the mean MAF results in dB re 0.0002 dyne/cm^2 for the men and women combined. The most important feature of the figure is the rapid increase in sound pressure levels necessary to reach the audible threshold as the sound frequency is increased above 12,000 Hz.

Figures 4.4 and 4.5 clearly indicate that the normal human ear is most sensitive to frequencies falling between about 1,000 and 4,000 Hz. At

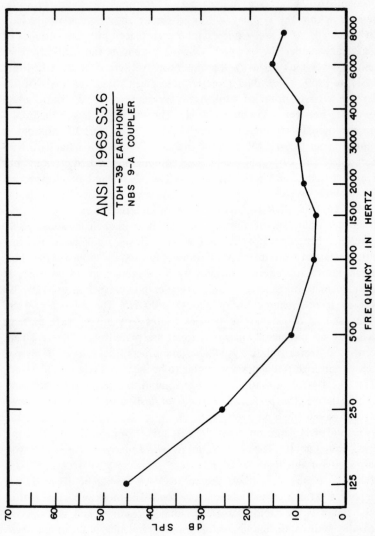

Figure 4.4. MAP reference thresholds. Courtesy American National Standards Institute. 1969. *Specifications for Audiometers.* S3.6.

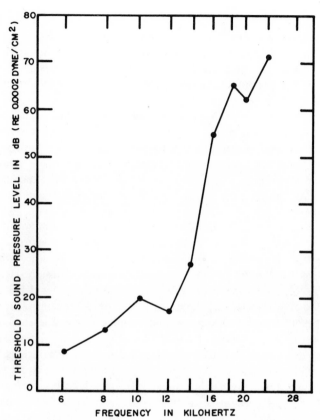

Figure 4.5. Audibility curve for 72 normal hearing young adults using the MAF method. From Corso, 1965.

frequencies which fall outside this range, the ear becomes less sensitive. The loss in sensitivity is particularly rapid for frequencies falling below about 250 Hz and above 12,000 Hz.

Experiment 1: Threshold Determination Using the Method of Limits

The present experiment is designed to illustrate the Method of Limits for determining the absolute threshold for tones. When determining the absolute threshold, the experimenter is, of course, concerned with finding that stimulus value which is capable of eliciting a response 50% on a number of trials. The physical measure used to determine auditory sensitivity, however, may vary. The measurement may be in decibels (e.g., dB re 1 dyne/cm^2, dB re 10^{-16} watt/cm^2, etc.) or may be in terms of voltage across the earphone terminals. In most instances in the clinic and laboratory, however, auditory thresholds are reported in dB SPL or in dB re some arbitrary voltage across the earphone terminals with no attenuation in the system. For purposes of illustration, both methods shall be employed in the present experiment. The test frequency is chosen to be 1,000 Hz.

To review briefly, the Method of Limits requires that the intensity of the stimuli be varied in alternating ascending and descending series. The series is composed of stimuli which are both above and below the assumed threshold level and which are distributed in equal increment steps. Furthermore, these steps in intensity are directly under the experimenter's control. An appropriate block diagram for the experiment is seen in Figure 4.6.

Equipment Arrangement An audio frequency oscillator set to 1,000 Hz serves as the input signal to an electronic switch. The electronic switch is controlled externally by an interval timer. The timer, in turn, is triggered by a manual pushbutton in the experimenter's room. Thus, the electronic switch in this arrangement serves only to control the rise and fall characteristics of the signals. The durations of the tones are controlled by the interval timer. The switch output is led through an amplifier, and then to the input of an attenuator. (It will be recalled that in Chapter 3 it was assumed that the impedances which existed between the various circuit components were matched. In actual practice, however, it is not uncommon for impedance mismatches to exist. Frequently, the input or output impedance of a laboratory instrument is 600 ohms while that of an output transducer is 10 ohms. Therefore, the following experimental apparatus arrangements shall require impedance matching at those circuit points where impedance differences often occur.) The output from the attenuator (Z = 600 ohms) is then led through an impedance matching transformer and into the subject's test room to a single earphone (Z = 10 ohms). A separate "ready" light system is also provided to alert the subject that a signal will be presented.

Calibration Before the actual calibration process is begun, it is of utmost importance that the investigator examine the interconnecting wires between the circuit components. This is to insure that the negative and positive circuit polarities have been observed. The initial step in calibration is to set the oscillator to 1,000 Hz. The oscillator frequency may be directly observed on a digital frequency counter. (Although frequency may be monitored at any point in the circuit, it is best to monitor directly at the oscillator output. At this point the frequency count will not be affected by the electronic switch operation or by the attenuator settings.)

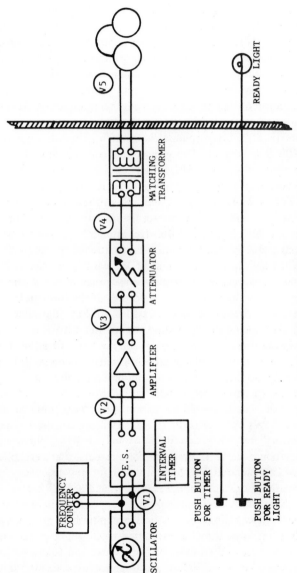

Figure 4.6. Block diagram for Method of Limits—Experiment 1.

The oscillator output voltage is then adjusted so that it adequately drives the electronic switch. This voltage (V_1) should remain constant for the remainder of the experiment. The electronic switch is the set to a "constant on" mode, or to a mode where the signal is on for a considerable length of time. For example, in the present arrangement, the interval timer may be set to deliver a 10-second tone. While the tone is on, the gain control on the electronic switch may be adjusted to deliver an adequate driving signal to the amplifier (the output waveform of the amplifier should be monitored while the input signal is being adjusted). At this point the attenuator is set to 0-dB attenuation. If the output signal is to be measured in dB SPL, the earphone may, at this time, be mounted in a standard NBS 9-A coupler. The gain control on the amplifier is set to produce an arbitrarily chosen SPL in the coupler. The voltage at point V_3 is recorded and must remain constant in order for the apparatus to remain calibrated. For example, 0.5 volt at point V_3 might produce an 80-dB SPL output at the earphone. If the apparatus is to remain in calibration (i.e., to always produce 80 dB SPL at 1,000 Hz) after the earphone is removed, point V_3 must always read 0.5 volt with no attenuation in the line. The voltage reading at V_4 will equal that at V_3 with zero attenuation. The voltage at V_5, however, will be slightly lower than V_3 or V_4 because of the insertion loss of the matching transformer. If the stimulus levels to be used in the test series are to be expressed in dB SPL, the values may be obtained by introducing an appropriate attenuation value.

As previously described, thresholds need not be reported in dB SPL. If a sound-level meter is not available, thresholds may be reported in dB re an arbitrary voltage applied across the earphone terminals. For example 0.3 volt across the earphone (with 0-dB attenuation) may be chosen as a reference voltage. The threshold for an individual would then be reported as $-X$ dB re 0.3 volt. As long as the reference voltage remains constant, the relative auditory sensitivity among individuals may be evaluated. (If a frequency response curve is available for the particular earphone being used, the SPLs generated by that earphone for any frequency may be closely estimated. For example, 0.5 volt may yield X dB SPL for 1,000 Hz and "Y" dB SPL for 4,000 Hz, and so on.)

Procedure   After calibration has been accomplished, the experimenter must decide upon those stimulus intensities which will be presented to the subjects. The stimulus values must lie both above and below the assumed threshold level. Therefore, before starting the experiment the experimenter must have some notion of where threshold is likely to be. If the subjects have normal hearing, the experimenter may choose the stimuli by referring to ANSI or ISO standards or the experimenter may choose to pretest a group of normal individuals. Table 4.5 shows a sample worksheet for determining threshold using the Method of Limits. Note that the stimuli are adjusted in 1-dB steps about the suspected threshold (about 7 dB SPL for 1,000-Hz tones according to both the ANSI and ISO standards).

An experimental session is initiated by placing the subject in a sound-treated test room. He is then instructed that a "ready light" will glow about 1.5–2 seconds before a tone presentation. The subject is told that he may or may not be able to perceive the tones which follow the light presentations. He is instructed to indicate whether or not the tone was perceived either vocally (using an intercom) or by vote buttons.

The tones in the present design are chosen to be about 2 seconds in duration. They are presented each time the experimenter triggers the interval timer manually using the push button. The ready light is also controlled manually.

Table 4.5. Sample worksheet for determining threshold using the Method of Limits

Stimulus frequency_____

Stimulus value in dB SPL	Asc.	Des.	Asc.	Des.	Asc.	Des.
14						
13						
12						
11						
10						
9						
8						
7						
6						
5						
4						
3						
2						
1						
0						

Series threshold

Overall mean threshold = _____ dB SPL

4.2. DIFFERENTIAL THRESHOLD MEASUREMENT

Classical Procedures

The use of the psychophysical methods is not only limited to the study of absolute auditory thresholds, but also may be extended to suprathreshold auditory measures as well. In particular, each of the methods may be used to determine the resolving power or discriminatory ability of the auditory system. The resolving power is the smallest physical difference between two stimuli which can be detected by an observer. This minimal difference is commonly referred to as the difference limen or the differential threshold. It has also frequently been called the just noticeable difference. Difference limens can be determined for many aspects of hearing. The most frequent investigations of DLs have sought the DL for intensity (DL_I) and the DL for frequency (DL_F). For example, the investigator may be interested in how the DL_I differs as the sensation level of a tone increases or he may be interested in determining how DL_F changes as the frequency is increased.

Difference limens have frequently been reported in two ways. The first is simply to report the absolute difference (ΔI or ΔF) between the standard stimulus and the stimulus which is judged to be just noticeably different from the standard. If DL_I is being sought for a 1,000-Hz tone at a sensation level of 40 dB, a tone which is just perceived as louder may have an SL of 42 dB. Thus, the absolute difference (ΔI) between the standard and the comparison judged just different is 2 dB. The second method of reporting DLs is in relative terms, where the absolute change required for one stimulus to be judged just noticeably different from another stimulus is divided by the value of the standard stimulus, i.e., $\Delta I/I$ or $\Delta F/F$. The fraction obtained when dividing the absolute increment by the standard is called the Weber fraction. In 1834 Weber pointed out that in order for one stimulus to be judged as just different from another stimulus, the absolute increment of the comparison stimulus must always be a constant proportion of the standard, i.e., $\Delta I/I = K$, where K is a constant value known as the Weber constant. A classic example of the testing of Weber's Law would be in an experiment to determine the DL for lifted weights. In such a study the observer might lift a standard weight to which additional weight would be added. The purpose of the study would, of course, be to determine the least increment in weight which would be detected by the observer. For example, one standard weight might be 90 grams to which weight increments of $\frac{1}{2}$ gram would be added. We might find that an addition of 3 grams would, on the average, be just noticeably different from the standard. Thus, the Weber fraction in this instance would be 0.03 ($\Delta W/W = \frac{3}{90} = 0.03$). To determine whether the Weber fraction remained constant with other standard weight values, the experiment would be repeated.

Considerable effort has been spent in determining the universality of Weber's Law for many sensory modalities. In general, it has been found that the Weber fraction does not remain constant over all stimulus values for any sensory dimension. This is particularly true when dealing with either the high or low standard magnitudes. At these extremes the Weber fractions tend to increase. This, of course, indicates a reduction in the discriminatory ability. The Weber fractions do remain relatively constant for many modalities in the middle intensity ranges.

As indicated previously, a threshold must be defined as a statistical value. This is because of the inherent variability of a given threshold from moment to moment. When dealing with the measurement of differential thresholds, the same relationship holds true. Therefore, an operational definition of the differential threshold is that stimulus value which is just perceived as being different from another stimulus 50% of the time.

When using the Method of Limits to determine the DL, the method is somewhat changed from that used to determine the absolute threshold. The underlying principle, however, is the same. That is, there are ascending and descending stimulus series about a reference point. When determining the absolute threshold, the reference point is the assumed threshold level. When determining the DL, the reference point is the standard stimulus value.

Determination of the DL using the Method of Limits requires that two stimuli be presented. The first stimulus, the *standard,* remains at a constant value throughout the investigation. The second stimulus, the *comparison,* assumes one of many values which are distributed in small increments about the standard. The comparison stimuli are presented in alternating ascending and descending series. To illustrate the procedure, a hypothetical experiment using the visual modality will be used. The experiment is designed to find the number of dots required to first perceive a difference in a standard dot field. The standard stimulus is chosen to be a random field of 30 dots. The comparison fields are randomly distributed fields of from 18–42 dots which vary in two-dot steps.

The standard field is presented for a given time interval (e.g., 3 seconds) followed by a comparison field presentation. As discussed, the comparison fields are presented in either an ascending or descending series. The subject's task is to indicate whether the comparison field is greater than (more dots), less than (fewer dots), or equal to (same number of dots) the number of dots in the standard field. Table 4.6 shows hypothetical results for the present dot numerosity study. The table shows that two DLs are calculated for each stimulus series. The upper DL corresponds to that point in each series where the judgment changes from equal (=) to greater than (+). The lower DL is that point in each series where the judgment changes from equal (=) to less than (−). Note that both the upper and lower DLs are considered to lie midway between the last negative (or positive) sign and the first equal sign. For example, in the first ascending series, the upper DL is recorded as three dots. This value represents the midpoint between the last equal sign (32 dots) and the first positive sign (34 dots). The absolute difference between the midpoint and the standard (three dots) is taken as the upper DL. Overall mean lower and upper DLs are calculated by averaging the six DL values. A grand, overall mean DL is also calculated. This latter value (3.34 dots) represents the overall resolving power of the task.

The *Method of Constant Stimuli* may also be used to determine a difference limen. The method used is similar to the Method of Limits in

Table 4.6. Calculation of the DL using the Method of Limits for a dot numerosity study

Comparison dot field	Asc.[a]	Des.	Asc.	Des.	Asc.	Des.
			Series type			
42			+			
40		+	+		+	
38	+	+	+	+	+	+
36	+	+	+	+	+	+
34	+	=	+	=	+	+
32	=	=	=	=	=	=
30 (St.)	=	=	=	=	=	=
28	=	=	=	=	=	−
26	−	−	−	=	−	−
24	−	−	−	−	−	−
22	−	−		−		−
20		−		−		
18		−				
Upper DL	3	5	3	5	3	3
Lower DL	3	3	3	5	3	1

[a]Asc., ascending; des., descending.
[b]Mean upper DL = 3.67 dots; mean lower DL = 3.00 dots; overall mean DL = 3.34 dots.

that the subject is presented with a standard and a comparison stimulus, but differs in that the comparison stimuli are presented randomly. In the variation of the Method of Constant Stimuli to be discussed, the subject is limited to either of two responses—greater or less. Thus, if the comparison appears to possess less of the attribute under investigation than the standard, a less (−) judgment is made. Conversely, if the comparison appears to possess more of the attribute than the standard, a greater (+) judgment is made. No equal judgments are permitted. As in the determination of the absolute threshold, about five to eight comparison stimuli are selected so that they range closely about the standard stimulus. Table 4.7 shows the results of a hypothetical experiment which is designed to determine the DL for lifted weights using the Method of Constant Stimuli.

In this study, the standard stimulus is chosen to be 200 grams. The comparison weights vary from 185—215 grams in 5-gram steps. In investigations of this type, where two stimuli are presented in succession, a bias

Table 4.7. Calculation of the DL using the Method of Constant Stimuli for a listed weights experiment

Trial	Constant stimuli in grams						
	185	190	195	(200)	205	210	215
1	−	−	+	+	−	+	+
2	−	−	+	+	+	+	+
3	−	+	−	−	+	+	+
4	−	−	−	+	−	+	+
5	−	+	−	−	+	+	+
6	−	−	−	−	−	+	+
7	−	+	−	−	+	+	+
8	−	−	−	−	−	+	3
9	−	−	+	+	−	+	+
10	−	−	+	+	+	+	+
11	−	−	−	+	+	+	+
12	−	−	−	−	+	+	+
13	−	+	−	−	+	+	+
14	−	−	+	+	+	+	+
15	−	−	+	−	+	−	+
16	−	−	−	−	−	+	+
17	−	−	+	−	−	+	+
18	−	−	−	+	−	+	+
19	−	−	−	+	+	−	+
20	−	−	−	+	+	−	+
Percent (+)	0	20	35	50	60	85	100
Percent (−)	100	80	65	50	40	15	0

known as *time error* may arise. This is so because the second stimulus is compared to a memory image of the first stimulus. It is not uncommon for a *negative time error* to occur, where the second stimulus is consistently overestimated because of the fading image of the first stimulus. To reduce bias, the experimental design may be counterbalanced by presenting the standard stimulus before the comparison on half the trials and the comparison stimulus before the standard on the remaining trials. As when using the Method of Constant Stimuli to obtain the absolute threshold, the comparison stimuli are presented in a random order. After each comparison stimulus has been paired with the standard a given number of times (20 judgments per comparison stimulus in the present example), the data may be summarized as shown at the bottom of Table 4.7. These values represent the percentage of the times that each comparison stimulus was judged either greater (+) or less than (−) the standard stimulus. As indicated, a subject is required to judge the second stimulus relative to the first. The subject is unaware, however, which stimulus is truly the standard and which one is the comparison because of counterbalancing. For data analysis the judgments must be made relative to the standard stimulus only. Therefore, in those trials where the standard came first in the pair, the judgments remain unaltered. However, in those trials where the comparison preceded the standard, the judgments must be reversed so that a plus response is scored as a negative, and vice versa. Table 4.7 is arranged so that the proper reversals have been made.

Figure 4.7 plots the percentage of "greater than" and the percentage of "less than" judgments for each of the comparison stimuli. These functions are mirror images of each other. To determine a DL from these psychometric functions, one must first consider that a comparison stimulus which elicits a "greater than" (or "less than") response 50% of the time is not being discriminated from the standard. In fact, one would expect this value on a chance basis. On the other hand, a comparison stimulus which is perceived 100% of the time as being "greater than" or "less than" is clearly being discriminated from the standard. The convention used to define the DL for this method is taken to fall midway between chance performance and perfect discrimination. Therefore, the 75% point on the curve plotting the percentage of "greater than" judgments, and the 75% point on the curve plotting the "less than" judgments, represent the upper and lower DLs, respectively. The upper DL in absolute terms is calculated by subtracting the weight which represents the 75th percentile on the "less than" function from the standard (8.3 grams).

The point at which both psychometric functions cross in Figure 4.7 is referred to as the point of subjective equality (PSE). It represents judg-

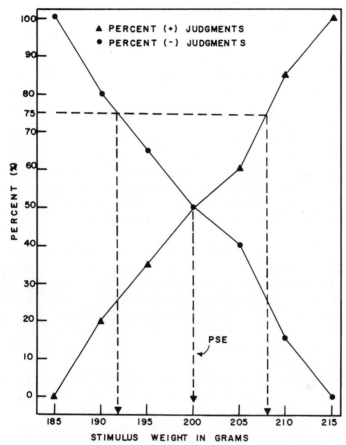

Figure 4.7. Psychometric function for DL determination using the Method of Constant Stimuli (hypothetical lifted weights data).

ments which are, on the average, subjectively equivalent to the standard. In this instance, the PSE is 200 grams.

The *Method of Average Error* may be used to determine the discrimination ability in a manner similar to that used in determining the absolute threshold. The subject is now presented with two stimuli, a standard and a comparison. The task is to adjust the magnitude of the comparison to equal the magnitude of the standard. Many judgments are made, and a mean setting of the comparison stimuli is calculated. The mean value of the comparison is called, once again, the point of subjective equality. The PSE minus the standard stimulus yields the CE, or constant error. The CE may be used directly as one index of discrimination. Another index of discrimination ability is the standard deviation of the comparison settings, which may also serve as the DL for the adjustment task.

Differential Thresholds for Frequency and Intensity

The DL is a measure of discrimination or acuity. It is an index of the least stimulus change necessary for one stimulus to be perceived as different from another. Two aspects of auditory acuity which have been investigated frequently have been frequency and intensity of pure tones. In frequency discrimination, the basic experimental problem is to hold intensity or loudness constant, to determine the least frequency separation between two tones which are perceived as different. In the case of intensity discrimination, the basic problem is to hold frequency constant, to determine the smallest intensive difference which is perceived as just different.

Harris (1952) determined frequency DLs for a wide range of frequencies (60–4,000 Hz) at various constant loudness levels (5–30 phons). A variant of the Method of Constant Stimuli was used to collect the data. Subjects listened to pairs of tones and were required to judge the second tone either "higher" or "lower" in pitch than the first tone (standard). Each tone in the pair was on for 1.4 seconds and separated by 1.4 seconds. A period of 4.2 seconds between the tone pairs permitted the subjects to record their answers.

Figure 4.8 shows how the difference limen for frequency varies as both a function of the frequency and loudness level of six test tones. Two important features are seen in the figure. As the loudness level decreases, there is an increase in the DL values. This increase is considerably more rapid at the higher test frequencies (particularly 4,000 Hz). The influence of loudness level, then, is less at the lower sound frequencies than it is when the frequency is raised. The second feature of the figure is that, for all frequencies, as the loudness level is increased, the DL values tend to stabilize.

Weber's Law states that, in order for one stimulus to be perceived as just noticeably different from another, a constant proportionality must exist between the standard and the comparison stimuli. In the case of frequency discrimination, $\Delta F/F$ should remain constant if Weber's Law were to hold. Figure 4.9 shows the absolute increments (in Hertz) shown in Figure 4.8 divided by the appropriate standard frequency. The calculated values are Weber fractions for each of the test conditions. These values may be used as a direct test of Weber's Law. Note that when the frequency effect seen in Figure 4.8 is eliminated by using these relative

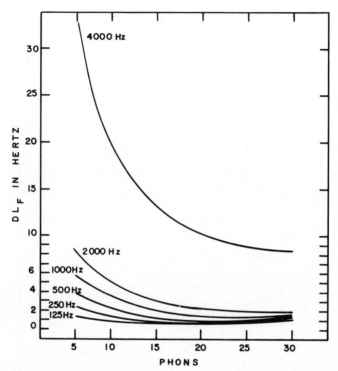

Figure 4.8. Difference limen for frequency in Hertz as a function of loudness level. From Harris, 1952.

measures, the relation between loudness level and DL remains relatively constant over a wide frequency range. In general, at low loudness levels, the obtained Weber fractions are considerably greater than those obtained as the loudness level is increased. As the loudness level is increased, there is a progressive decrease in the Weber fractions until the values appear to level off at about 20–25 phons. Shower and Biddulph (1931), in their classic paper dealing with frequency DLs found, as Harris (1952) observed later, that the Weber fraction remained relatively unchanged at sensation levels above about 40 dB.

Riesz (1928) investigated the difference limen for intensity using a method in which the outputs of two audio frequency oscillators were mixed. The frequencies of the oscillators were set 3 Hz apart so as to produce a single intermediate tone whose amplitude fluctuated at a rate of 3 Hz/second. The subjects were asked to judge whether the tone sounded constant in loudness or whether it fluctuated in loudness. The DL_I was taken as that intensity level at which the fluctuations were first perceived.

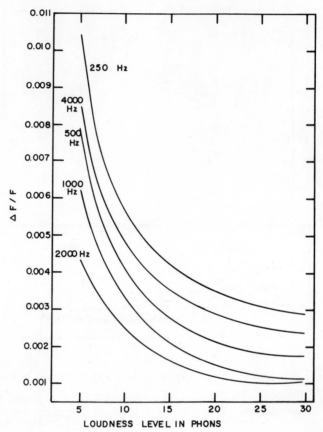

Figure 4.9. Difference limen for frequency in ΔF/F as a function of loudness level. From Harris, 1952.

Figure 4.10 shows the obtained DLs in absolute (ΔI in dB) and relative (ΔI/I) terms as a function of the sensation level of various test frequencies. Two relations are evident from the figure. First, for each test frequency, as the SL is reduced, there is a considerable increase in the obtained DL values. Thus, at low SLs, we are relatively less responsive to sound intensity increases than at higher sensation levels. Secondly, at SLs of about 40 dB and higher, ΔI/I remains relatively constant. Figure 4.11 replots the data in Figure 4.10 so that the relative DL_I (ΔI/I) is plotted against frequency for seven sensation levels. The figure shows clearly that intensity discrimination at low frequencies is considerably less acute than at higher frequencies when the tones are of low sensation level. However,

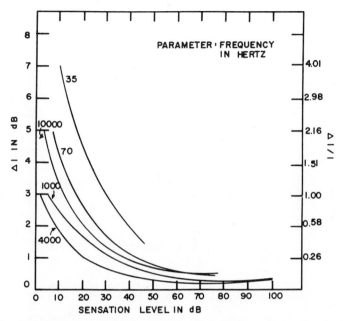

Figure 4.10. Difference limen for intensity as a function of sensation level for various frequency tones. From Riesz, 1928.

as the SL is increased, the low frequency DLs improve rapidly relative to the higher frequency DLs. This improvement is so rapid that, at SLs of about 40 dB and greater, the acuity for all test frequencies is nearly equivalent.

Experiment 2:   Determination of the Difference Limen for Frequency Using the Method of Constant Stimuli

The present experiment is designed to determine the DL_F for a tone at a given sound pressure level. In the example given, the standard tone is 1,000 Hz at 40 dB SPL. A block diagram of the experimental apparatus is shown in Figure 4.12.

Equipment Arrangement   The equipment consists of two oscillators whose output frequencies are alternately presented to a single earphone. This is accomplished by first taking the output from oscillator 1 and feeding it to the input of an electronic switch. The output from oscillator 2 is then led to the input of a second electronic switch. In this particular design, the on-times of the tones are externally controlled by interval timers. The interval timers, in turn, are capable of turning each other on

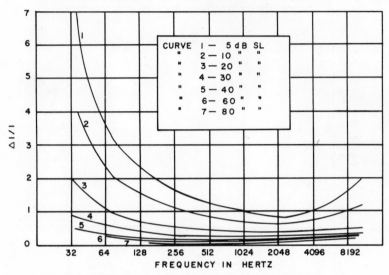

Figure 4.11. Difference limen for intensity as a function of frequency. The parameter of the figure is sensation level. From Riesz, 1928.

and off. The outputs from the electronic switches feed separate amplifiers which, in turn, are led to individual attenuators. The attenuator outputs are then electronically mixed. To this point, all the input and output impedances are matched at 600 ohms. As in the previous design, the output transducer is assumed to be 10 ohms. Therefore, an impedance-matching transformer is interposed between the mixing network and the earphone.

Calibration   Before actually discussing the calibration process, it is worthwhile to briefly review the Method of Constant Stimuli. The method calls for two stimuli to be presented in succession. One stimulus is the standard value. The other stimulus represents one of several comparison stimuli which closely range about the standard. The subject's task is to judge whether the second stimulus in the pair possesses more or less of the attribute under investigation than the first stimulus.

When seeking to determine the difference limen for frequency, it is imperative that the sound levels in both channels equal each other. This, of course, is to reduce the possibility of a bias arising from unequal intensity levels which might influence the frequency discrimination process. The calibration process insures that both channels are of equal levels.

The calibration process is similar to those presented in Figures 3.5 and 3.6 in that each channel is calibrated separately. To ensure independence

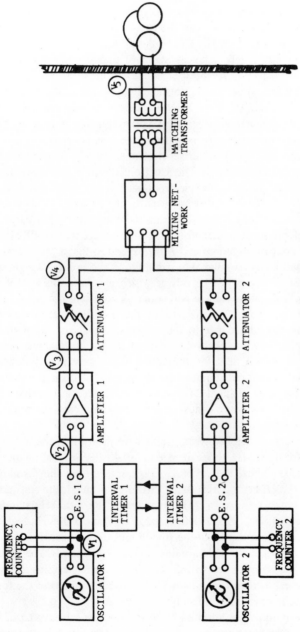

Figure 4.12.   Apparatus arrangement for DL$_f$ experiment.

of the channels during the calibration procedure, the attenuator of the opposite channel should be adjusted to maximum attenuation. The initial step in the calibration of channel 1 (upper channel) is to set the frequency of oscillator 1 to 1,000 Hz. In this design the outputs of both channels 1 and 2 will alternately serve as standard and comparison stimuli. (The calibration frequency for both channels will be 1,000 Hz. The frequency response of the apparatus is presumed to be flat in the small frequency range to be used (994–1,006 Hz). Therefore, only one calibration frequency per channel is necessary.) This frequency is read on frequency counter 1. The output voltage from the oscillator should be set to a sufficiently high level to drive electronic switch 1. This voltage (V_1) should remain unchanged. The electronic switch may now be set to a "constant on" position. The electronic switch gain control is then adjusted to provide an adequate driving signal to the amplifier. This voltage (V_2) should also remain unchanged during the experiment. The earphone may now be placed in an artificial ear, and attenuator 1 set to 0-dB attenuation. The gain control on amplifier 1 is then raised so that a predetermined SPL is generated in the coupler. For example, in the present design, a level of 100 dB SPL is chosen. The voltage which produces this level is noted at point V_3. This latter voltage will equal V_4, but will not equal the voltage across the earphone (V_5) because of the insertion loss produced by the mixer and the impedance matching transformer. For the equipment to remain in calibration, the voltage at points V_4 or V_5 must remain constant. The desired SPL for the actual experiment may be obtained by inserting an appropriate amount of attenuation (60 dB in this instance).

Calibration of channel 2 (lower channel) is identical to that of channel 1 except that attenuator 1 must be set to maximum attenuation before the calibration process.

Procedure   Previous investigations have shown that the Weber fraction ($\Delta F/F$) for 1,000-Hz tones at a level of 40 dB SPL is, on the average, about 0.003. Thus, the absolute DL for this frequency is about 3 Hz (0.003 $\times$ 1,000 Hz = 3 Hz). With this value in mind, the constant stimuli can be chosen to vary in 2-Hz steps about the 1,000-Hz standard. The values are 994, 996, 998, 1,000, 1,002, 1,004, and 1,006 Hz.

The timing sequences of the stimuli must now be set. It is decided that both tones in the pair will have durations of 1.5 seconds. The time interval between the tones is set to 0.5 seconds. An interstimulus interval of 10 seconds separates each tone pair. The rise- and fall-times of the tones is set to 25 msec in order to avoid audible transients.

The experiment is initiated by instructing the subject that he will hear two tones which are separated by a short time interval. Both tones will be heard in one ear only. The subject is further told that he is to judge the second tone relative to the first as higher or lower in pitch.

Since both channels of the apparatus alternate as standard and comparison, the experimenter must have a prearranged schedule of the frequencies to be presented in a pair. The standard frequency (1,000 Hz) will simply alternate between channels on successive trials. The comparison frequencies will also alternate, but will change randomly. Table 4.8 shows a segment of a presentation program which might be presented to a subject. The total number of pairs to be presented (N) is equal to the number of constant stimuli multiplied by the number of trials each constant stimulus is to be judged. In the present experiment, it is decided to pair each comparison stimulus 20 times with the standard. Therefore, a total of 140 judgments will be made. (A relatively long ISI has been included in the experimental design to allow the experimenter time to set the appropriate frequencies between judgments. If the experimenter desires to monitor the presented signal aurally, a second earphone of equivalent impedance may be placed in parallel with the test earphone. This may

Table 4.8. Segment of a presentation program to be judged by a subject in Experiment 2

Pair number	First stimulus	Second stimulus
1	1,000 Hz[a]	998 Hz
2	992 Hz	1,000 Hz
3	1,000 Hz	1,006 Hz
4	998 Hz	1,000 Hz
5	1,000 Hz	1,006 Hz
6	1,000 Hz	1,000 Hz
7	1,000 Hz	996 Hz
8	992 Hz	1,000 Hz
9	1,000 Hz	1,002 Hz
10	998 Hz	1,000 Hz
11	1,000 Hz	996 Hz
12	1,000 Hz	1,000 Hz
13	1,000 Hz	998 Hz
14	992 Hz	1,000 Hz
15	1,000 Hz	1,002 Hz
.	.	.
.	.	.
.	.	.
N[b]		

[a]All tones = 40 dB SPL.
[b]N = total number of stimulus pairs to be judged.

reduce the SPL in the test earphone to a certain extent. To recalibrate, place the test earphone in the coupler and set the appropriate attenuator to 0-dB attenuation. Increase the amplifier gain until the original SPL is obtained. Note the new voltage and recalibrate the opposite channel in the same way.)

The stimulus pairs may now be presented to the subject who will record his judgments on an answer sheet. Table 4.9 shows a sample worksheet for sorting the data obtained from the subject's answer sheet. Note that each constant stimulus value has been paired with the standard 20 times. When recording the responses, the experimenter must consider that the subjects have judged the second stimulus relative to the first stimulus in all instances. The subjects were not aware of which tone was, in actuality, the standard or comparison. The judgments to be recorded in Table 4.9 must be relative to the standard stimulus only. Therefore, for those pairs where the standard tone preceded the comparison tone, the judgments may be recorded as reported by the subject. For those pairs where the standard tone followed the comparison, the judgments are reversed.

The upper, lower, and overall means DLs are computed in the manner previously described.

4.3. LOUDNESS AND PITCH PERCEPTION

The loudness of a sound represents the psychological percept of intensity. Therefore, the terms *loudness* and *intensity* should not be confused. The loudness-intensity dichotomy exists primarily because human observers do not generally judge loudness on a purely physical basis as would be expected. As will be seen later in this section, a doubling of loudness, on the average, corresponds to about a 10-dB intensity difference between two stimuli. The 10-dB difference would not be expected if loudness were judged purely on physical quantity. When physical intensity (in dB SPL) is doubled (or halved), the dB difference between the two sounds is only 6 dB (i.e., $N_{dB} = 20 \log 2/1 = 20 (0.3) = 6$ dB).

The pitch of a sound represents the psychological percept of frequency. Therefore, the terms *pitch* and *frequency* should not be confused. As in the case of loudness perception, human observers do not judge pitch on a purely physical basis. For example, if the frequency of two pure tones were set one octave apart (e.g., 1,000 and 2,000 Hz) and presented to an observer, the judged ratio between the two sounds would not be 2:1. In the case where the two tones are 1,000 and 2,000 Hz, the 2,000 Hz tone will, on the average, be judged about 1.5 times as great in pitch as the

Table 4.9. Sample worksheet for determining DL_F using the Method of Constant Stimuli

Trial no.	Constant stimulus value in Hz						
	994	996	998	1,000 (St.)	1,002	1,004	1,006
1	.	.	.	.	. .	.	.
2	.	.	.	.	.	.	.
3	.	.	.	.	.	.	.
.							
.							
.							
20	.	.	.	.	.	.	.
Percent (+)							
Percent (−)							

1,000 Hz tone (Stevens and Volkmann, 1940). Thus, the dichotomy between pitch and frequency must be observed.

Scaling Sensations

A goal of any science is to quantify the various relations under investigation. This quantification, of course, requires a scale of measurement. Measurement, however, may be made at different levels. It ranges from the simple classification of different items into separate categories to more complex relations dealing with ratios between various items on the scale. Psychophysics, like any other science, is concerned with measurement, and different psychophysical problems lend themselves to different levels of measurement. Four types of scales are used in psychophysical measurement: nominal, ordinal, interval, and ratio. The purposes and uses of these scales are well known (Stevens, 1951).

The *nominal* scale represents the simplest level of measurement because only the classification of attributes is considered without regard to ordering. Several psychophysical problems lend themselves to measurement using nominal scales. Foremost among these are the determination of both absolute and differential thresholds. In the former case the subject is simply required to classify his judgments into one of two categories—"Yes, the stimulus is present" or "No, the stimulus is not present." In a similar manner, when measuring the differential threshold, the subject is required to judge between those stimuli which are different from or not different from the standard. The *equation of magnitudes* is another area in psychophysics which is measured using a nominal scale. In these experiments, the subject judges whether or not one stimulus appears to be equivalent in some aspect to another stimulus. For example, in determining equal loudness contours (to be discussed), the subject is required to judge whether or not one tone is equivalent in loudness to another tone.

Ordinal scales are one step removed from nominal scales in that they arrange things in order. These scales, however, are not designed to indicate the distance between two attributes.

Interval scales are another step removed from nominal scales in that the distance between two scale values may be determined with precision. These scales, however, do not possess true zero points. A true zero point represents that there are no attributes under investigation. For example, the centigrade scale arbitrarily sets a temperature of $0°C$ as the freezing point. This temperature, however, is not a true zero point because temperature extends well below this value. A ruler, on the other hand, does have a true zero point because there is a true zero inches point.

Ratio scales represent the most advanced measurement scales in that they contain an interval scale within themselves and have true zero points. The most important aspect of ratio scales is that one scale quantity may be related to other scale values in terms of a ratio. For example, in the case of the ruler, the true zero point allows us to say that one distance is twice or half as great as another.

Ratio scaling techniques have been developed which seek to quantify subjective sensations. That is, these methods permit psychophysical scales to be developed which preserve information about ratios between sensations. These methods have been used in the scaling of both loudness and pitch perception. Generally, four ratio scaling procedures have been used: Magnitude Estimation, Magnitude Production, Ratio Estimation, and Ratio Production.

Magnitude Estimation refers to the method in which subjects assign numbers to each stimulus in a stimulus series. Each judgment represents a numerical estimation of the psychological magnitude of the stimulus. Two Magnitude Estimation procedures are used frequently. The first method requires that an arbitrary number (modulus) be assigned to the first stimulus in a stimulus pair. The first stimulus (standard) always assumes the same stimulus value, but the second stimulus (comparison) may assume one of many values along the continuum under investigation. The subject's task is to estimate the sensation of the comparison stimulus relative to the modulus number assigned to the standard. In the second procedure, no modulus is included and the subject reports his subjective impressions by any number which he feels is directly proportional to the stimulus magnitude.

Magnitude Production is the inverse of Magnitude Estimation. In this method the subject adjusts a variable control to produce subjective sensations which are proportional to numbers suggested by the experimenter. The method of Magnitude Production has been used in conjunction with Magnitude Estimation as a combined method known as *Numerical Magnitude Balance* (Hellman and Zwislocki, 1963).

Ratio Estimation is a method in which the experimenter chooses two stimuli and then asks the subject to assign a ratio between them. For example, the experimenter might present two tones which are 10 dB apart and then require the subject to judge the perceived loudness ratio between them.

In *Ratio Production* the subject is required to produce a prescribed ratio between two stimuli. In one form of Ratio Production, *Fractionation,* the subject is presented with a standard stimulus and is asked to adjust a variable stimulus to some fraction (usually one-half) of the standard. In another form of Ratio Production (*Multiple Stimuli*) the subject is asked to adjust the comparison stimulus to some multiple of the standard. Typically, the multiple is twice the standard.

Psychophysical Scales of Loudness and Pitch

Loudness Scales The earliest psychophysical loudness scales were based upon Ratio Production methods, principally the Method of Fractionation. Churcher (1935) brought together the results of several studies which had investigated loudness relations using the Fractionation procedure where one tone was judged half the loudness of another tone of the same frequency. He found considerable agreement among these studies and was able to construct an overall psychophysical loudness scale from the data. To do this, he arbitrarily assigned the value "100" to the loudness of a 1,000-Hz tone at a level of 100 dB HTL. The stimulus value which, on the average, was judged half of the 100-dB HTL tone was assigned the scale value of "50." The stimulus level judged half of the value corresponding to "50" was then assigned the scale value "25," and so on. Stevens (1936) reasoned that loudness scales would be used extensively by many professionals and, therefore, it was appropriate to define the fundamental unit of loudness. Just as any standard unit of measurement (e.g., feet, pounds, etc.) must be precisely defined so that measurements are repeatable from location to location, so was it true of loudness measurements. The unit of loudness chosen by Stevens (1936) was the *sone*. He defined 1 sone as the loudness of a 1,000-Hz tone at a level 40 dB above threshold (40 dB SL).

Loudness scales may be erected in a number of ways. One procedure is to base the scale solely upon fractionation data. A second procedure would be to use a combination of the Methods of Fractionation and Multiple Stimuli. This latter procedure will presently be used to illustrate the steps in erecting a sone scale of loudness.

To begin with, the experimenter must define his basic measurement unit. The unit in this instance is a 1-sone tone (i.e., the loudness of a 1,000 Hz at 40 dB SL). To determine the intensity level associated with a 2-sone tone (that tone which sounds twice as loud as a 1-sone tone), the subject is presented with two stimuli. The subject's task is to adjust the level of the comparison tone to twice the loudness of the standard 1-sone tone. This intensity level is assigned the value 2 sones. To determine the intensity level associated with a 4-sone tone, or that level at which the tone sounds twice the loudness of a 2-sone tone, the subject is once again presented with a stimulus pair. The level of the comparison is adjusted to twice the loudness of the standard (which is now set to the level associated with 2 sones). This process is continued until the stimulus level reaches about 100–110 dB SPL. To erect the scale at values below 1 sone, the Method of Fractionation is used. For example, a 0.5-sone tone may be obtained by having the subject adjust the comparison stimulus to one-half the loudness of a 1-sone tone. The stimulus level associated with the 0.5-sone tone then becomes the standard stimulus for determination of a 0.25-sone tone. This process is continued to a level near the audible threshold.

In the Ratio Production procedures, the experimenter prescribes the sensation ratio to be set by the subject. The opposite of Ratio Production then is Magnitude Estimation, where the subject is free to specify the subjective ratio between stimuli.

Stevens (1956) presented loudness scales which were erected using the two variants of the Method of Magnitude Estimation. In the method using a modulus, observers were presented with stimulus pairs. The first stimulus in the pair (standard) was always set to 80 dB SPL and was assigned the loudness "10" by the experimenter. The second stimulus in the pair assumed one of nine levels which covered a 70-dB range (30–100 dB SPL). The comparison tones were presented in a random order. All tones were 1,000 Hz. The subject's task was to estimate the loudness of the comparison stimulus relative to the assigned value of the standard. In the second variation, no modulus was designated and no restrictions were placed upon the subject's mode of responding. Eight tones (1,000 Hz) were spaced in 10-dB steps from 40–110 dB SPL. Each of these tones was presented to each subject twice in a random order. The subjects were asked to indicate the loudness of each tone by assigning it a number which they felt was directly proportional to the subjective impression. Since each subject used a modulus of his own choice, the data for the subjects were brought into coincidence by multiplying by an appropriate factor.

Figure 4.13 shows the results obtained by Stevens (1956) for both variants of the Method of Magnitude Estimation. Also shown in the figure is the sone scale as recommended by the International Standards Organization (ISO R131-1959; *Expression of the Physical and Subjective Magnitudes of Sound or Noise*). The values associated with the sone function may be read from the right-hand ordinate, while the magnitude estimates may be read from the left-hand ordinate. The median magnitude estimates obtained by Stevens (1956) for judgments made with a modulus are shown by the filled circles, and those made without a modulus are shown by the triangles. The data obtained for both variants may be well fitted by a single line which is also shown in the figure.

The most important feature of Figure 4.13 is that, although the two plotted functions are slightly displaced from each other because of the different reference points, both the ISO and the magnitude estimation functions are straight lines and have identical slopes. This similarity of function is important because, if the phenomenon of loudness perception is to be fully understood, the relations between sound pressure and subjective sensation should remain invariant across measurement methods.

The functions plotted in Figure 4.13 tell us much about loudness perception. Stimulus magnitude and judged loudness are related by a linear (straight line) function when plotted on logarithmic coordinates. (Even though the abscissa in Figure 4.13 is linear, decibels are logarithmic units. In fact, both axes are logarithmic.) Therefore, perceived loudness approximates a *power function* of stimulus intensity. The reader will recall that a power function is a straight line on log-log coordinates. The meaning of the power function is that equal stimulus ratios correspond to equal subjective ratios. In the case of loudness, the slope of the power function is such that every doubling (or halving) in judged loudness is associated with about a 10-dB difference in stimulus intensity. The latter relation is sometimes known as the "10-dB rule" (Stevens, 1957a).

The fact that loudness perception is a power function of stimulus intensity is of considerable theoretical interest because such functions can be found for at least a dozen other perceptual continua (Stevens, 1957b). These continua include brightness perception, visual distance, taste, dura-

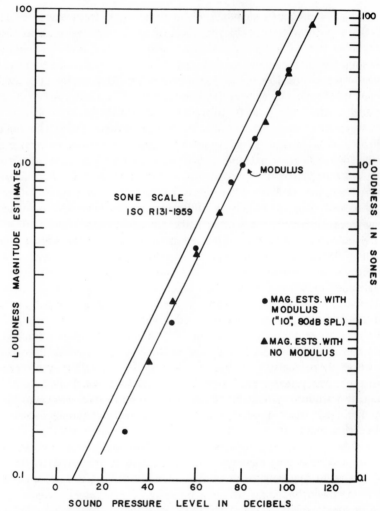

Figure 4.13. Psychophysical loudness scales obtained by Stevens (1956) and the Sone scale adopted by ISO (1959). See text for details.

tion, heaviness, and visual flash rate, among others. Thus, the power function for loudness appears to be one instance of what Stevens (1957*b*) has called the general "psychophysical law." It should be noted that the slope (exponent) of the power function varies with the modality under investigation. The slope of the loudness power function is 0.6 for sound pressure and 0.3 for sound power.

Pitch Scales Psychophysical scales of pitch (i.e., those scales which relate subjective pitch to frequency) have been established using the Method of Fractionation. As in loudness perception, an arbitrary unit of sensation has been established. This unit is called the *mel,* and 1,000 mels are equivalent to the pitch of a 1,000-Hz tone at a loudness level between 55 and 60 phons (Stevens and Volkmann, 1940).

One of the earliest studies to quantify the relation between pitch and frequency was that of Stevens, Volkmann, and Newman (1937), who used the Method of Fractionation. These investigators presented 10 standard frequencies between 125 and 12,000 Hz to their subjects. The subjects' task was to adjust a variable frequency control to one-half the pitch of the standard. From the obtained mean data points, one-half-pitch functions were plotted. These functions were used to establish the mel scale in a manner which will be specified later in the present chapter.

Stevens and Volkmann (1940) used the Method of Fractionation to examine further the frequency-pitch relation. Eight standard frequencies ranging from 150–10,000 Hz were used. A standard tone was presented for 2 seconds, followed immediately by a 2-second comparison tone. The frequency of the comparison tone could be adjusted by the subject. Both the standard and comparison tones remained at a loudness level of about 55 phons. The subject's task was to adjust the pitch of the comparison tone to one-half that of the standard. Thus, the procedure used in this study closely paralleled that used in the earlier 1937 study. However, one difference was present. The subject could, whenever he desired, turn a knob to introduce a 40-Hz tone. The subjects were told that this tone approximated "zero" pitch and that the fractionations should be made with that in mind.

Figure 4.14 shows the Mel scale obtained by Stevens and Volkmann (1940). The most important aspect of the figure is that pitch perception is not related to fequency in any simple manner. For example, a pitch of 2,000 mels, which is twice the apparent pitch of 1,000 mels, corresponds to a frequency of 3,000 Hz. A pitch of 500 mels corresponds to a 400-Hz tone, while a pitch of 250 mels corresponds to a 300-Hz tone.

The loudness scales plotted in Figure 4.13 and the pitch scale plotted in Figure 4.14 show a fundamental difference in that while the loudness scale may be represented as a power function of stimulus intensity, the Mel scale assumes a curvilinear form. Thus, loudness adheres to the general psychophysical law (Stevens, 1957*b*) and the pitch function does not. Stevens (1957*b*) has noted that perceptual continua divide themselves into two categories. Class I, or prothetic, continua represent sensations which are mediated by additive processes at the physiological level. Class II, or

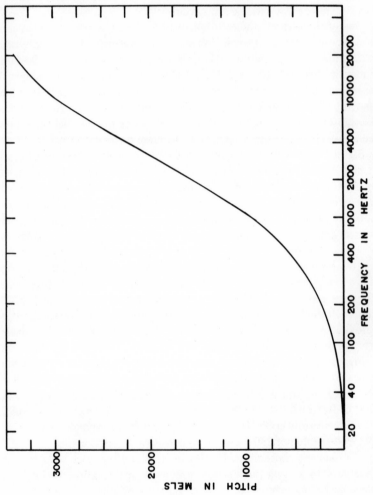

Figure 4.14. Psychophysical Mel scale for pitch perception. From Stevens and Volkmann, 1940.

metathetic, contunua represent sensations that are mediated by substitutive processes at the physiological level (i.e., sensations which change because of differences in the locus of excitation). In general, sensations which are governed by prothetic processes, such as loudness perception, produce psychophysical scales which are power functions of stimulus magnitude and which agree with the general psychophysical law. This law does not hold on metathetic continua such as pitch.

Experiment 3: Psychophysical Scale of Loudness
Using the Method of Magnitude Estimation with a Modulus

Loudness scaling has frequently been accomplished using the Method of Magnitude Estimation with a modulus. To reiterate, the modulus represents a standard stimulus to which the experimenter assigns an arbitrary number. The experimenter then presents other stimuli which are paired with the modulus. These other stimuli are both above and below the intensity of the modulus. The task of the subject is to assign a number to the comparison stimuli relative to the number assigned to the standard. The subject is free to choose any numbers he feels are appropriate to represent the magnitudes of the comparison stimuli. Figure 4.15 shows a block diagram of the equipment used to obtain a subjective scale of loudness using the above method.

Equipment Arrangement The present arrangement is similar to that used in Experiment 2 except that the output from one oscillator is split and fed to the inputs of both electronic switches. This arrangement insures that the standard and comparison tones will not differ in frequency. The output from the oscillator (1,000 Hz in the present experiment) is alternately presented through both electronic switches to a single earphone. As in the previous design, the on-times of the tones are governed by the interval timers. The interval timers, in turn, are mutually wired so that they control each other. The outputs from the electronic switches feed their respective amplifiers and attenuators. The outputs are then mixed and feed the earphone via an impedance-matching transformer. In this design, channel 1 (upper circuit) serves as the standard stimulus channel, and channel 2 (lower circuit) serves as the comparison stimulus channel. Note that both attenuators are within the experimenter's control room.

Calibration After the frequency of the oscillator has been set to 1,000 Hz, each channel is calibrated separately. An adequate driving voltage to both electronic switches is set using the oscillator gain control. This voltage (V_1) is to remain unchanged. If channel 1 is to be calibrated first, attenuator 2 is set for maximum attenuation. Attenuator 1 is then set for minimum (0-dB) attenuation, and the earphone placed in the artificial

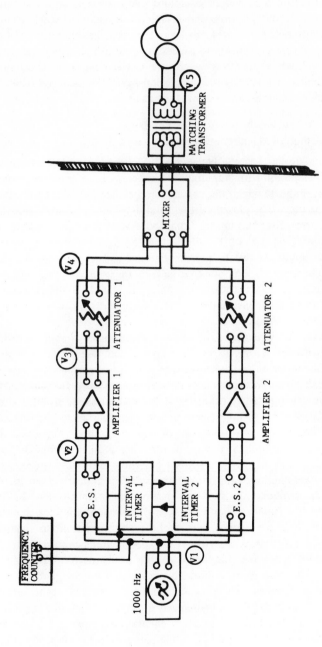

Figure 4.15. Experiment 3 block diagram.

ear assembly. The output of electronic switch 1, which should now be in a "constant on" mode, is set to adequately drive amplifier 1. This voltage (V_2) should remain unchanged. The amplifier gain is now adjusted to yield a predetermined sound pressure level in the coupler. In this instance the output is set to 100 dB SPL. The voltage which produces this SPL is noted at either points V_3, V_4, or V_5 (the voltage at V_5 should be somewhat lower than at the other two points) and should remain constant in order to maintain calibration. The same process is repeated for channel 2 with attenuator 1 set at its maximum attenuation point.

The modulus in the present design is chosen to be 70 dB SPL. The comparison stimuli vary from 40–100 dB SPL in 10-dB increments. Therefore, to produce the desired SPL for the modulus 30-dB, attenuation must be introduced into the standard channel using attenuator 1. The comparison stimuli levels may be obtained by introducing appropriate attenuator values using attenuator 2. Table 4.10 shows the attenuation settings to be used for the comparison stimuli when 0-dB attenuation yields 100 dB SPL at the test earphone.

After the calibration process has been completed, the timing parameters may be set. It is decided that the standard tone (modulus) will be presented for 1.5 seconds followed 0.5 seconds later by a 1.5-second comparison tone. A 5-second interval follows in which the subject records his responses. The next standard-comparison pair is then presented.

Procedure The subject is seated in an adjacent room or may be seated in the same room as the experimenter if quiet conditions prevail. The subject is instructed that he will hear pairs of tones and that the task will be to judge the loudness of the second tone relative to the loudness of the first tone. The subject is further told that the loudness of the first tone will not change, but that the loudness of the second tone will. The

Table 4.10. Attentuation values that yield comparison stimuli between 40 and 100 dB SPL (0-dB attenuation = 100 dB SPL)

Comparison stimulus in dB SPL	Attenuator 2 setting
100	0
90	10
80	20
70	30
60	40
50	50
40	60

loudness of the first tone is assigned the number "10." The subject is free to choose whatever numbers he feels represent the subjective magnitudes of the comparisons relative to the modulus number.

The comparison stimuli are presented in a random order. In the present experiment it is decided that each subject will make three magnitude estimates for each of the seven comparison stimuli. A minimum of 10 subjects will be used in the study. All subjects should have normal hearing.

Table 4.11 shows hypothetical results for the present study. Each value in the table represents the median magnitude estimate for one subject when judging a given comparison tone. An overall median is also computed for each comparison tone. These later values are used in erecting the loudness scale.

Before plotting the loudness scale from the data in Table 4.11, it is worthwhile to examine closely the meaning of the mean magnitude estimates in the table in terms of loudness perception. Note that the 70-dB SPL comparison stimulus was assigned the subjective magnitude "10." Since the modulus was 70 dB SPL and assigned the value "10," this equivalence in subjective sensation might be expected. The 80-dB SPL comparison tone was assigned the median magnitude estimate "20," indicating that the tone sounded twice as loud as the modulus. The 60-dB SPL stimulus, on the other hand, was assigned the subjective magnitude "5." This indicates that the 60-dB SPL tone sounded one-half the loudness of the modulus.

Table 4.11. Hypothetical magnitude estimates for 10 subjects

	Comparison stimuli in sound pressure level						
Subject	40	50	60	70	80	90	100
1	1	3	8	9	21	25	83
2	1.5	2	5	10	18	35	100
3	2	7	5	10	17	40	75
4	3	1	7	11	20	45	80
5	1	5	5	12	20	40	80
6	1	2	4	10	20	40	80
7	0.5	2	5	8	15	35	50
8	0.9	3	6	10	21	50	65
9	1	3	8	10	20	40	82
10	2	2	5	10	20	45	80
Overall median magnitude estimate in dB SPL	1.3	2.5	5	10	20	40	80

Figure 4.16 plots the hypothetical median magnitude estimates shown in Table 4.11 as a function of their respective sound pressure levels. The plotted values may be well fitted by a straight line. Therefore, the results of the hypothetical experiment show loudness to be a power function of stimulus intensity. The slope of the line is such that each 10-dB increment in intensity is associated with a 2:1 loudness ratio. Thus, this hypothetical

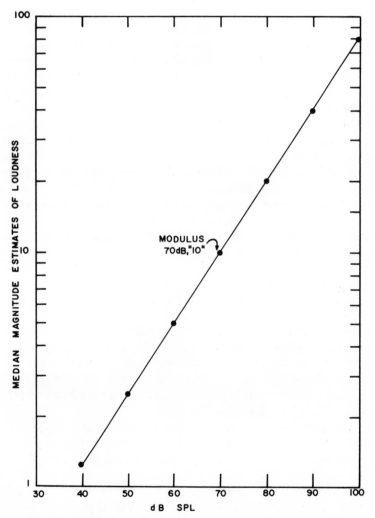

Figure 4.16. Hypothetical magnitude estimates function for loudness plotted from the median magnitude estimates in Table 4.11.

function adheres to the "10-dB rule" discussed previously. The reader should be well aware that the data shown here are purely hypothetical. They have been chosen only to illustrate certain relevant points. Departures from these values *are* to be expected in actual experimentation.

Experiment 4: Psychophysical Scale of Pitch
Using the Method of Fractionation

The Method of Fractionation differs from that of Magnitude Estimation in that the subject is allowed to adjust the second (comparison) stimulus to some prescribed ratio of the standard. For example, the subject's task might be to adjust a variable attenuator so that the comparison stimulus is one-half the magnitude of the standard. A psychophysical scale of pitch may be obtained in this fashion. To this end, it is first necessary to first choose an arbitrary unit of pitch and to assign a frequency to it. The arbitrary unit used frequently in pitch scaling is the mel, and the value 1,000 mels is equated to the subjective pitch of a 1,000-Hz tone set at a loudness level of between 55 and 60 phons. Before discussing the actual procedure to be used in the experiment, it is necessary that the student fully understand the experimental paradigm. Using the Method of Fractionation, a standard tone is first presented. This is followed by a comparison tone of an equivalent loudness level. The subject cannot change the frequency of the standard, but can adjust the frequency of the comparison.

The procedure which is commonly used in erecting a Mel scale, or any other psychophysical scale based upon the Method of Fractionation, is to first choose several standard stimulus points which traverse the physical continuum under investigation. The task of the subject is to fractionate these standard stimuli in a manner specified by the experimenter (i.e., one-half judgments). The outcome of this fractionation procedure yields data which may be plotted as a half-magnitude function, or a function which relates the magnitude of the standard stimulus to the magnitude of the stimulus judged half. The psychophysical scale is then erected from this function in the manner specified below.

To illustrate the procedure, a fictitious physical unit will be used. The unit is called a *pol*. The pol may be the stimulus necessary to stimulate any sense modality. To initiate the study, the experimenter should choose pol values which traverse the modality from near threshold levels to relatively high stimulus levels. The following values are chosen: 20, 40, 60, 80, 100, 120, 140, 160, and 180 pols. Each of the standard pol values are then presented to the subject(s) in an A-B sequence, where A is the standard stimulus and B is the comparison stimulus. The task is to adjust the comparison stimulus to one-half the magnitude of the standard. The standard stimuli are presented randomly, and the subject makes a number of half judgments for each standard. Once the data have been collected they may be arranged as seen in Table 4.12.

Table 4.12 shows the median one-half pol values obtained for each subject for each standard. Thus, each cell in the table may represent five judgments for each standard pol value. An overall median one-half judgment is obtained for each standard value. Once the data have been arranged, as in Table 4.12, a half-magnitude function may be plotted. Figure 4.17 shows the function which relates the standard pol values to the pol values judged half.

To erect the psychophysical scale, it is necessary to choose an arbitrary unit of sensation and to equate it to some pol value. The sensation unit is arbitrarily called a *sen* (for *sen*sation), and the value 1,000 sens is equated to 100 pols. Figure 4.18 shows the psychophysical sen scale, i.e., a scale which relates the physical stimuli, pols, to its psychological percept, reported in units called sens. This scale is constructed directly from the information in Figure 4.17.

Point 1 on Figure 4.18 represents the arbitrary reference point chosen for the scale. Thus, 100 pols are equated to 1,000 sens. Point 2 on the scale represents 500 sens and corresponds to that stimulus value which was judged half the subjective magnitude of the 1,000-sen standard. This stimulus value may be obtained directly from Figure 4.17. It corresponds to 66 pols. Thus, 66 pols is assigned the subjective value of 500 sens. Point 3 in Figure 4.18 represents a 250-sen value or that sensation which is judged half the magnitude of the 500-sen stimulus. Since 500 sens cor-

Table 4.12. Half-magnitude judgments for each of the standard pol values

Subject	Standard pol value									
	20	40	60	80	100	120	140	160	180	200
1	15	25	45	61	71	75	107	105	125	120
2	25	32	48	52	63	82	94	136	130	145
3	20	25	35	49	66	91	88	141	145	150
.	.	.	.	.	.	.	.	.	.	.
.	.	.	.	.	.	.	.	.	.	.
.	.	.	.	.	.	.	.	.	.	.
N	18	20	30	63	65	84	115	101	107	135
Median one-half pol value	15	26	40	52	66	80	100	120	130	140

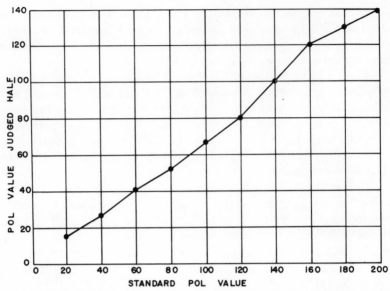

Figure 4.17. Half-pol function relating standard pol values to those pol values judged half.

responds to a stimulus value of 66 pols, a 250-sen value is that stimulus level judged half of 66 pols. Referring to Figure 4.17, it is seen that the stimulus judged half of 66 pols is 43 pols. Thus, the stimulus 43 pols is assigned the value of 250 sens and plotted accordingly. Point 4 on Figure 4.18 is 125 sens, or that sensation judged half of 250 sens. To determine the stimulus value associated with 125 sens, it is necessary that half the subjective magnitude of the 250-sen signal be determined. Referring, once again, to Figure 4.17, the value judged half of 43 pols (250 sens) is 28 pols. This latter point is plotted accordingly. Point 5 on Figure 4.18 is plotted in the same fashion as points 2–4.

Those points which lie above the 1,000 sen, 100-pol standard are also plotted using the half-pol function. Point 6 represents a subjective value of 2,000 sens, or that sensation which is judged twice the magnitude of the standard. To obtain this point the experimenter must determine what intensity was judged twice the 100-pol standard. Referring to Figure 4.17, it is seen that 100 pols is judged one-half the magnitude of 140 pols. Point 7 represents that magnitude which is 4,000 sens, or twice the apparent magnitude of 2,000 sens. Since 2,000 sens equals 140 pols, it must be determined which stimulus value appears twice 140 pols. Figure 4.17 indicates that this value is 200 pols. Thus, 200 pols is assigned the subjective magnitude of 4,000 sens.

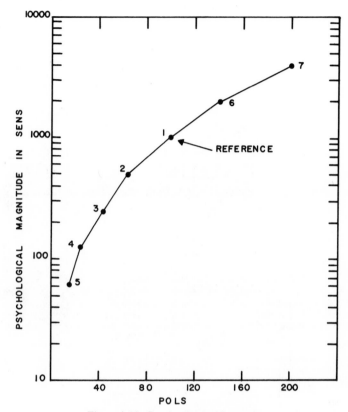

Figure 4.18. Psychophysical Sen scale.

A Mel scale is generated in much the same manner as the hypothetical Sen scale. A number of standard frequencies are presented to the subject. The subject is then required to fractionate the standards using a variable frequency control. A half-pitch function is plotted from which the Mel scale may be erected.

Figure 4.19 shows an appropriate block diagram for the pitch scaling experiment.

Equipment Arrangement The equipment arrangement is similar to those presented in previous experiments. The apparatus alternately presents the frequencies of two oscillators. In this design, however, the frequency of oscillator 2 is directly uder the subject's control, while the frequency of oscillator 1 (standard) is under the experimenter's control. The conditions present in each facility will dictate the arrangement to be used in providing the subject control of the oscillator. Probably the simplest way of having the subject control the frequency of the oscillator

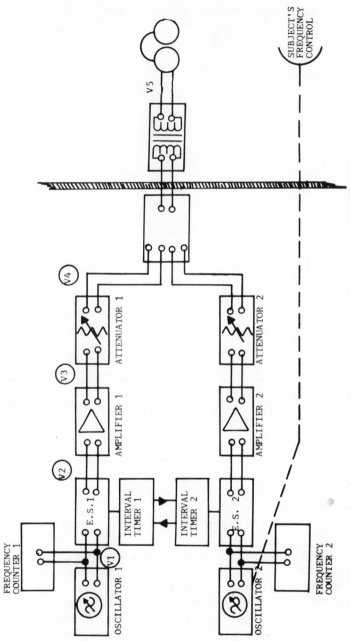

Figure 4.19. Equipment arrangement for pitch scaling Experiment 4.

is to place oscillator 2 in the subject's test chamber, or the experimenter might decide to mechanically couple the tuning dial to a long shaft which extends into the subject's test chamber. In any event, the subject's oscillator should be capable of traversing a large frequency range without bandswitching. Therefore, it is advantageous to provide the subject with the dial of a beat frequency oscillator. The face of the oscillator should be obscured so as not to provide any cues for the judgments. Frequency counter 2 should be placed in the experimenter's room.

Calibration   Calibration of the intensities in the present experiment is somewhat more complex than in the previous experiments. This complexity arises because the loudness of the standard and comparison tones should remain unchanged. This is to avoid any possible biasing effects caused by sound intensity on the perception of pitch. The loudness level used here will be approximately 60 phons for all tones.

The Mel scale in this experiment is based upon eight standard frequencies: 250, 500, 1,000, 2,000, 3,000, 4,000, 6,000, and 8,000 Hz. The standard tones are presented using channel 1 (upper half of the circuit), while the comparison tones are presented using channel 2 (lower half of the circuit).

Figure 4.20 shows the 60-phon equal loudness (isophonic) contour presented by Robinson and Dadson (1956). This function serves as a reference in calibrating both circuit channels in the present study.

To calibrate channel 1, first set oscillator 1 to 1,000 Hz. Electronic switch 1 should now be set to a constant on condition. Attenuator 2 should be set at maximum attenuation. The oscillator 1 output voltage (V_1) is then set to drive the electronic switch. This voltage, of course, should now remain constant. As in the previous designs, the electronic switch output is adjusted to provide an adequate working voltage to the amplifier (V_2). Attenuator 1 is then set to 0-dB attenuation, and the gain on amplifier 1 adjusted so that a predetermined SPL is produced at the earphone. This voltage is noted at either points V_3, V_4, or V_5, and should remain unchanged. In the present experiment the output SPL is chosen to be 100 dB SPL.

Since all the standard tones are to be presented at a given loudness level, it is now necessary to determine the attenuation settings which produce sound pressure levels which correspond to 60 phons at each of the standard frequencies. This may be accomplished by referring to the isophonic contour presented in Figure 4.20. For example, a 60-phon tone at 1,000 Hz represents a 60-dB SPL stimulus level. Therefore, for the average observer (the Robinson and Dadson (1956) study was based upon normal hearing individuals), 40-dB attenuation is necessary to produce the 60-

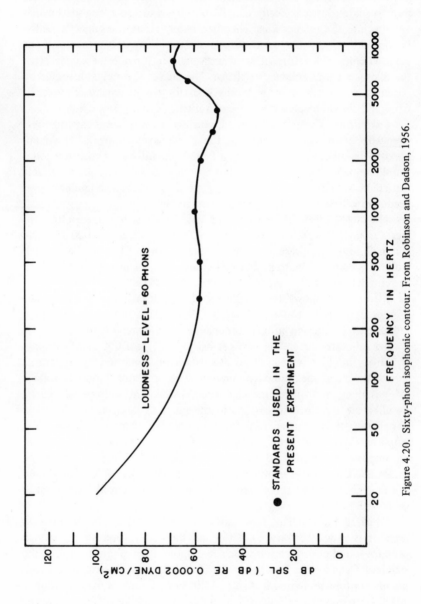

Figure 4.20. Sixty-phon isophonic contour. From Robinson and Dadson, 1956.

phon loudness level. This attenuation value is noted. To obtain the 60-phon level at the other standard frequencies, the frequency is changed and the output SPL is observed (attenuation = 0 dB). For example, the output at 250 Hz may read 102 dB SPL. (The earphone's frequency response may alter the output SPL relative to the 1,000-Hz tone. This, however, will not interfere with the calibration process.) Figure 4.20 shows that a 60-phon loudness level at 250 Hz corresponds to a tone at 56 dB SPL. Therefore, it is necessary that 46 dB of attenuation be introduced using attenuator 1 whenever a 250-Hz tone is used as the standard. This process is continued until the attenuation values have been determined for all the standard tones.

Although it is relatively easy to calibrate the phon levels for each of the standard frequencies, it is impossible to calibrate each and every comparison frequency that the subject hears when performing his frac- tionations. Therefore, the convention adopted is to calibrate various fre- quencies and, as the subject approaches these calibration frequencies, to adjust attenuator 2 to a preset attenuation point. A tone located in the general frequency region should then approximate a level of 60 phons. The calibration frequencies to be used are the same as the standard tones.

The calibration process for channel 2 is the same as that for channel 1 except that attenuator 1 must be set to maximum. The phon levels are calibrated in exactly the same manner as described above. If this is done properly, the attenuation values which produce the required 60-phon levels for channel 2 should be nearly identical to those obtained for channel 1.

After calibration of both channels has been completed, the timing parameters may be set. It is decided that the standard tone will be presented for 2 seconds. This will be followed by 0.50 second of silence and then a 2-second comparison tone. A 4-second interval will separate each stimulus pair.

Procedure The experimenter instructs the subject that he will hear pairs of tones which are separated by a short time interval. The subject is also told that he will not be able to control the pitch of the first tone but will be able to control the pitch of the second tone using the knob (to oscillator 2) in front of him. The task is to adjust the pitch of the second tone to one-half the pitch of the first tone. The subject is informed that the tone pairs will be repeated after 4 seconds and that he may use as many sequences as necessary to feel fully satisfied with his judgment.

The experimenter may begin with any standard frequency. During the judgmental process, frequency counter 2 should be monitored, and the attenuation values on attenuator 2 adjusted accordingly. After the subject has made his judgment, another standard is presented. The standards should, of course, be presented in a random order. In this experiment, five half-pitch judgments for each standard frequency for each subject will be obtained. Table 4.13 shows how the data may be arranged. Each entry represents the median half-pitch judgment for each of the subjects for each standard frequency tone. A grand median half-pitch value is calculated for each standard. These data are plotted as a half-pitch function which, in turn, is used to plot the Mel scale. The scale itself may be erected in a manner directly analogous to the method used to plot the Sen scale earlier in the chapter.

Equal Loudness

Loudness relations for tones may be investigated in two principle ways. In one instance, the frequency of the test stimuli are held constant and the intensity levels are varied. This is the method used in loudness scaling, where the loudness associated with one sound is compared to the loudness associated with another sound of the same frequency. The second way of investigating the loudness of tones is to perform loudness balances between tones of differing frequency. In this way the effect of frequency upon loudness becomes apparent.

In their classic study, Fletcher and Munson (1933) suggested that 1,000-Hz reference tones be used when performing loudness matches between frequencies. They further suggested that the *loudness level* of these reference tones be specified in units called "phons," the number of phons being numerically equal to the dB SPL of the 1,000-Hz tone. Thus,

Table 4.13. Half-pitch judgments for eight standard frequencies

Subject	Standard frequency in Hz							
	250	500	1,000	2,000	3,000	4,000	6,000	8,000
1	.	.	.	.	.	.	.	.
2	.	.	.	.	.	.	.	.
3	.	.	.	.	.	.	.	.
.								
.								
.								
N	.	.	.	.	.	.	.	.
Overall median one-half pitch value in Hz	.	.	.	.	.	.	.	.

a 1,000-Hz reference tone at a level of 50 dB SPL would have a loudness level of 50 phons, and a 1,000-Hz reference tone at 75 dB SPL would have a loudness level of 75 phons. The loudness level (in phons) of any other frequency would then be equivalent to the intensity in dB SPL of a 1,000-Hz tone judged equally loud. For example, if one tone sounded as loud as a 1,000-Hz tone at 60 dB SPL, the loudness level of the comparison tone would be 60 phons.

Fletcher and Munson (1933) had listeners perform equal loudness balances between 1,000-Hz reference tones and 10 comparison frequencies which ranged from 62–16,000 Hz. The reference intensities varied over a 120-dB range. All measurements were made under free-field conditions with the observer facing the sound source.

Some years later, Robinson and Dadson (1956) investigated equal loudness on a more extensive scale than the earlier study. They increased both the frequency and intensity ranges of the stimuli and used a large number of otologically normal subjects. Their frequency range extended from 25–15,000 Hz and their intensity range extended up to 130 dB SPL. Listeners were placed in an anechoic chamber and were faced directly toward the sound source. The Method of Constant Stimuli was used to obtain the loudness balance judgments.

Figure 4.21 shows the results obtained by Robinson and Dadson (1956) in the form of *equal loudness contours.* Each contour is identified by the phon value of the 1,000-Hz reference tone. For example, the 60-phon contour represents those sound pressure levels necessary for tones of other frequencies to sound equally loud as the 60-phon reference tone. Similarly, the 100-phon contour represents those sound pressure levels necessary to achieve equal loudness between the 100-phon standard (1,000 Hz at 100 dB SPL) and tones of other frequencies.

The most important feature of Figure 4.21 is that as the loudness level increases, the effect of frequency on loudness judgments decreases. That is, the contours for the higher loudness levels are considerably flatter than those obtained at the lower loudness levels. Consider, for example, the 20- and 120-phon contours. Observation of the 20-phon contour shows that a tone of 100 Hz must be raised to about 40 dB SPL in order to produce a loudness level of 20 phons. Thus, the difference between the standard tone (1,000 Hz at 20 dB SPL) and the comparison is about 20 dB. When the reference tone is raised to 120 phons, however, the equal loudness point for a 100-Hz tone is 125 dB SPL, or a 5-dB difference between the standard and the comparison.

As the reader might well know, in most instances it is impossible to perform equal loudness experiments under ideal free-field conditions.

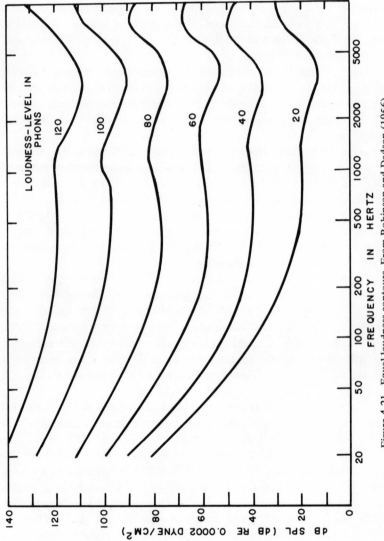

Figure 4.21. Equal loudness contours. From Robinson and Dadson (1956).

However, these experiments may be performed quite adequately using calibrated earphones. Thus, the loudness matches may be obtained by presenting the standard and comparison tones in sequence to the same ear or by presenting the standard to one ear and the comparison to the other.

Figures 4.22 and 4.23 show two block diagrams for equipment arrangements which may be used to obtain loudness matches using the Method of Adjustment. In the first circuit the standard 1,000-Hz tones are presented to one ear while the comparison tones are presented to the opposite ear. In the second circuit, both the standard and comparison tones are presented to one ear. Note that in both instances the subject adjusts attenuator 2. Attenuator 1 is used by the experimenter to set the standard intensity levels. Calibrations of both the upper and lower halves of the circuits in both figures are similar to those presented previously in Experiments 3 and 4. A suggested timing sequence might be to have the standard tone on for a period of 2 seconds, then 0.5 seconds of silence, and then a 2-second comparison tone. The subject's task is to adjust his attenuator so that the standard and comparison tones are of equivalent loudness.

Relation of Pitch to Sound Intensity

Pitch perception is primarily dependent upon the frequency and, to some extent, on the intensity of test tones. The Mel scale has shown perceived pitch to be monotonically related to frequency. Sound intensity changes do influence pitch, although not to the extent advocated by earlier investigations.

Stevens (1935) presented the most well-known set of functions relating pitch to intensity. In this study the observer was presented with alternating standard and comparison tones. The standard tones ranged from 150–12,000 Hz and had loudness levels between 30 and 100 phons. The comparison tones were set to slightly different frequencies than the standard tones. The subject matched the pitch of the comparison to that of the standard by adjusting the intensity of the comparison tone. The results showed that the effect of increased stimulus intensity was 1) to raise the pitch of the high frequency tones, 2) to lower the pitch of low frequency tones, and 3) to have a negligible effect on the pitch of the middle frequency tones.

The relations found by Stevens (1935) were not fully substantiated in subsequent investigations (Morgan, Garner, and Galambos, 1951; Cohen, 1961). These latter studies agreed with Stevens' results in that they too found that, as intensity was increased, pitch fell at lower frequencies and rose at higher frequencies. However, the extent of these pitch changes was

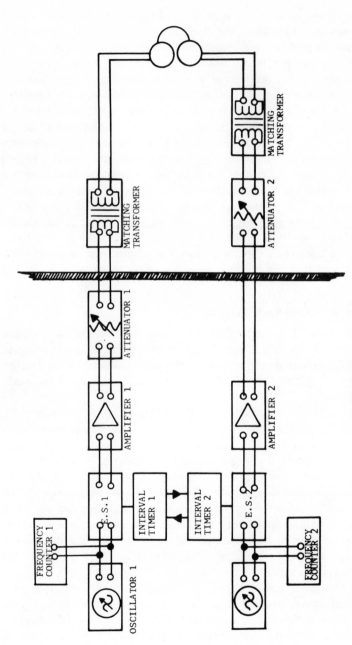

Figure 4.22. Loudness matches in two ears.

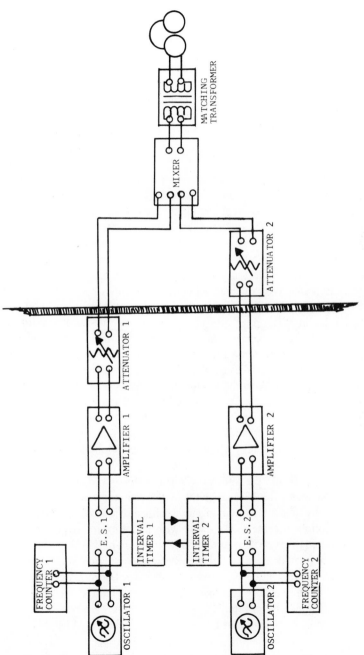

Figure 4.23. Loudness matches in one ear.

considerably less than the changes obtained in the 1935 study. The discrepancies have been attributed to differences in methodology among the studies and also to Stevens' use of only one experimental subject.

Cohen (1961) performed two experiments to investigate further the intensity-pitch relation. In the first experiment pitch changes were noted for frequencies between 50 and 6,000 Hz as each tone was raised from 40 to 100 phons. In the second experiment pitch changes were observed for tones between 100 and 6,000 Hz as each tone was raised in loudness level from 30 to 90 phons. The experimental paradigms for both experiments are seen in Figure 4.24. For the sake of simplicity, other control conditions used by Cohen (1961) are omitted from the figure. The reader is referred to the original article for complete details. In both experiments subjects made pitch matches between standard and comparison tones. The standard tones were set at one of four loudness levels (40, 50, 60, or 70 phons in Experiment 1 and 30, 50, 70, or 90 phons in Experiment 2). The frequency of the standard tone remained unchanged. The comparison tones were set at a fixed loudness level (40 phons in Experiment 1 and 30 phons in Experiment 2) and were variable in frequency.

Those test conditions in Experiment 1 where the standard tones were set to a loudness level of 40 phons served as the baselines for the evaluation of pitch changes associated with the other test conditions. Similarly, when the standard tones in Experiment 2 were set to 30 phons, the obtained results served as baselines for evaluating pitch changes for the remaining conditions. A modified Method of Limits was used to obtain the pitch matches. The method consisted of two ascending and two descending trials in which the frequency of the comparison tone was varied. The frequency steps in these trials were equal to the DL_F for the particular standard tone under study. All pitch matches were obtained under monaural conditions.

Figure 4.25 shows the results of Cohen's (1961) study. The abscissa of the function shows the loudness level of the standard tones. The ordinate was arbitrarily chosen so that a curve with an upward (positive) slope showed a pitch increase and a curve with a downward (negative) slope showed a pitch decrease. The amount and direction of the pitch change for any frequency is taken as the difference between the obtained percentage values at the lowest and progressively higher phon levels for the frequency of interest. With regard to this figure, Cohen (1961) noted that the effects of increased intensity on pitch were similar to those observed by Stevens (1935). That is, as the stimulus intensity was increased, the higher frequencies rose in pitch while the lower frequencies dropped in pitch. These changes, however, were markedly less than those obtained by Stevens in

	STANDARD TONE IN HZ	STANDARD LOUDNESS LEVEL	COMPARISON TONE FREQUENCY	COMPARISON TONE LOUDNESS LEVEL
EXPERIMENT I	50 Hz 75 Hz 100 Hz 150 Hz 200 Hz 1500 Hz 6000 Hz	40 Phons 50 Phons 60 Phons 70 Phons	"X"	40 Phons
EXPERIMENT II	100 Hz 200 Hz 400 Hz 700 Hz 1500 Hz 6000 Hz	30 Phons 50 Phons 70 Phons 90 Phons	"X"	30 Phons

Figure 4.24. Cohen's paradigms for determining pitch-intensity relations. From Cohen (1961).

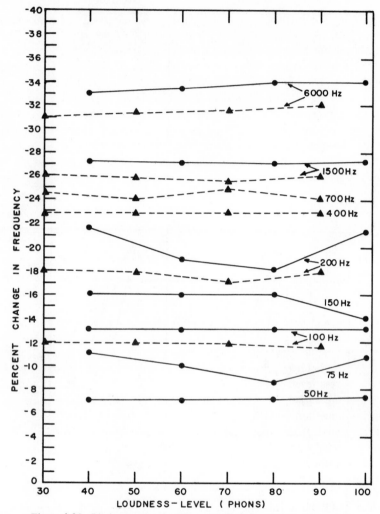

Figure 4.25. Pitch-intensity functions. From Cohen (1961; Figure 5c).

the earlier study, with the effect of increased intensity changing pitch, on the average, by 2% or less.

Morgan, Garner, and Galambos (1951) investigated the pitch-intensity relation for frequencies between 125 and 8,000 Hz and for intensity levels to 100 dB SPL. Two experimental methods were used. The first, the "anchor" method was somewhat similar to that used later by Cohen (1961). In this method, the intensity of the standard was set to 40 dB

SPL, while the intensities of the comparison tones varied in 10-dB steps. This is just the reverse of the method used later by Cohen (1961). The subject adjusted the frequency of the comparison tone so that it matched the pitch of the standard tone. The second method, the "ladder" method, always kept the standard tone at 10 dB below the level of the comparison tone. After the pitch match was made, both tones were raised 10 dB.

The experimental results showed that both the "anchor" and "ladder" methods yielded essentially the same results. Therefore, the data were pooled. Morgan, Garner, and Galambos (1951) reported a great deal of variability in the pitch-matching results among their subjects. Therefore, they sought central tendencies for their data rather than reporting data for individuals. The results of these analyses showed, in line with Cohen's (1961) findings, that the median change in pitch never exceeded 2%, although there was a tendency for low tones to decrease in pitch and for high tones to increase in pitch with increased intensity level.

An appropriate equipment arrangement for investigating pitch-intensity relations may be seen in Figure 4.19. The circuit arrangement seen in Figure 4.19 lends itself readily to pitch matching using the Method of Adjustment. That is, the frequency dial of oscillator 2 is directly under the subject's control while the intensity levels of both the upper and lower channels are under the experimenter's control. If the reader desires to use the experimental paradigm used by Cohen (1961) (Figure 4.24), the lower half of the circuit (comparison channel) is set to a constant loudness level. The loudness levels presented by the upper half of the circuit (standard channel) are varied. If, on the other hand, the reader wishes to use the "anchor" method used by Morgan, Garner, and Galambos (1951), the intensity level of the upper channel remains constant (40 dB SPL), while that presented by the lower channel varies. In both instances, however, it is the frequency of the lower channel which is varied to obtain the pitch matches.

Relation of Pitch to Duration

To this point in the discussion of pitch perception, it has been assumed that the tones are presented for an appreciable time period, i.e., for at least 0.25 second. Doughty and Garner (1947) reported that the pitch of a tone burst goes through three stages. In the first stage, where the burst duration is very brief, only a click is heard. As the duration is increased the tone assumes some tonal character (click-pitch threshold). In the third stage the tone assumes a definite tonal character (tone-pitch threshold) which does not change with further increases in duration. Figure 4.26 shows the click-pitch and the tone-pitch thresholds as a function of frequency. Two

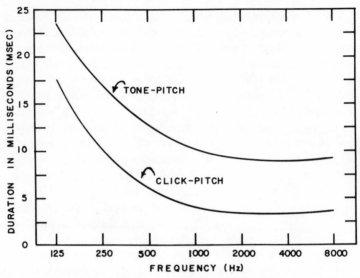

Figure 4.26. Tone-pitch and click-pitch. Relation between frequency and tone dura-tion for two types of pitch sensation. From Doughty and Garner (1947).

relations are evident. The first is that the two functions are displaced from one another as would be expected. Secondly, tones of lower frequency (below 1,000 Hz) require a greater duration burst in order to acquire a tonal character. In the region where the ear is most sensitive (1,000–4,000 Hz) the thresholds for both click-pitch and tone-pitch are shortest in duration.

4.4. TEMPORAL SUMMATION

It is well established that a functional relation exists between the duration of acoustic stimulation and auditory behavior. That is, the expenditure of acoustic energy will not produce a response unless it is expended over some minimum length of time. The reciprocal relation between time and intensity has frequently been referred to as auditory *temporal summation* or *integration.* The present section is concerned with various aspects of this psychoacoustic phenomenon.

Temporal Summation at the Audible Threshold

Perhaps the most thoroughly investigated aspect of auditory temporal summation is the relation which exists between stimulus duration and the threshold of audibility. Although this relation is not simple, it may generally be stated that, as one decreases stimulus duration below about 200 msec (sometimes referred to as the "critical duration"), an increase in stimulus intensity is required to maintain the threshold response. At durations above this point, the intensity necessary to maintain the threshold remains relatively unchanged. Thus, the temporal summation phenomenon for threshold responses is generally confined to durations below about 200 msec ($\frac{1}{5}$ second).

If the ear were to act as a perfect integrator of acoustic energy, where the threshold level was exactly inversely proportional to changes in stimulus duration, then the following relation would hold:

$$I \times t = k$$

In this equation, I is the stimulus intensity, t is the stimulus duration, and k is the threshold energy. Such a perfect trading relation would predict that every 10-fold (decade) decrease in duration would require a 10-fold increase in sound energy (10 dB) to maintain the threshold level. For example, if a tone were to be reduced in duration from 200 msec to 20 msec (a 1-log-unit decrease), it would require a 10-dB increase (a 1-log-unit increase) in energy in order to maintain the threshold level.

Garner and Miller (1947) investigated temporal summation at threshold using pure tones at 250, 1,000, and 4,000 Hz and white-noise. Thresholds were determined for durations between 1 msec and 100 msec using the Method of Limits. The results of the study showed that the above reciprocal relation did not hold for either the white-noise or the 250 Hz tones. In the former instance, the slope of the temporal summation function (i.e., the function relating duration to threshold level—both coordinates are plotted logarithmically) was only 8 dB/decade time decrease. In the latter instance, the slope of the function approximated 10 dB/decade time decrease until the very shortest tones where the function became less steep.

Garner and Miller (1947) recognized the limitations of the simple reciprocal model of temporal summation at threshold. Therefore, they modified it. Their modification may be expressed by the relation:

$$t\,(I - I_o) = k$$

where t is the stimulus duration, I is the stimulus intensity, I_o is a portion of the signal intensity which the ear cannot use, and k is the threshold energy. In effect, the model states that there is a minimal intensity (I_o) above which the ear will summate energy in a perfectly linear manner (i.e., the temporal summation function will change at a rate of 10 dB/decade decrease in duration), but below which summation will not occur. Licklider (1951) has called this model the "diverted input hypothesis" because a constant portion of the stimulus power is diverted from the summation process.

Olsen and Carhart (1966) investigated the temporal summation process for 250-, 1,000-, and 4,000-Hz tones and for white-noise. The durations of the tones were 10, 20, 50, 100, 200, 500, and 1,000 msec. A tracking task was used to obtain the threshold values. Subjects were instructed to push a switch in one direction to attenuate the signals and to push the switch in the opposite direction to increase the signal levels. The recording attenuator was placed in a step mode condition where the signals either increased or decreased in 1-dB steps.

Figure 4.27 shows the temporal summation functions obtained by Olsen and Carhart (1966). The functions have been plotted so that the threshold levels for the various stimulus durations are referenced to the 1,000-msec threshold for each stimulus type. The abscissa is plotted in terms of the *equivalent duration* of the test stimuli (the concept of equivalent duration will be fully discussed below). The most important feature of the figure is that for stimulus durations between 50 and 1,000 msec the curves are all similar. This indicates that the temporal summation process is relatively unaffected by stimulus type. At durations below 50 msec, however, the functions do exhibit some differences. In particular, the threshold for 250-Hz tones increases more rapidly than the other frequencies at durations of 10 and 20 msec. These differences were found to be statistically significant. The reason governing this divergence is believed to rest in the fact that the spread of energy for short-duration tones at 250 Hz is wider than the critical bandwidth for that frequency. Since the summation process is believed to occur only within the critical band, some of the energy in the tone burst is not used, and, therefore, additional energy is necessary to reach the threshold level. This increases the slope of the temporal summation function. The Olsen and Carhart (1966) results agree well with the model proposed by Garner and Miller (1947).

A special physical problem is encountered when tones of finite duration are used, particularly when the tone durations are as brief as those employed in temporal summation studies. The problem arises because if a tone is turned on or off abruptly (i.e., instantaneous rise- and fall-times) certain other frequency components (transients) will be introduced along with the frequency of interest. For short tones this spread of energy is related to the tone duration, with the bandwidth of the energy surrounding the frequency of interest being generally defined as $\pm 1/t$, where t is the burst duration (Garner, 1947). For example, if a 2,000 Hz tone burst

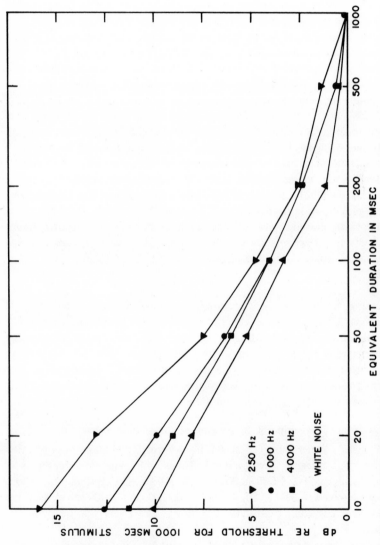

Figure 4.27. Mean increase in stimulus intensity required for threshold response as the signal is decreased in duration from 1,000 msec. From Olsen and Carhart (1966).

has a duration of 10 msec (0.01 sec), the main energy band surrounding the 2,000 Hz tone will drop off from a maximum energy level near 2,000 Hz to zero energy levels at approximately 1,900 Hz and 2,100 Hz. In addition to the main energy band surrounding the 2,000 Hz tone other continuous frequency bands, both above and below the main, occur.

The spreading of energy to unwanted frequencies results in an audible click or thump. The subject may respond to the click and not to the tonal sensation when making a threshold judgment, and, thus, the experimental results will be biased. The problems introduced by transients at the beginning and end of tone bursts may be effectively reduced by altering the rise- and fall-times of the stimuli. For most applications (such as in pure tone audiometric testing), the process of altering the rise- and fall-times of signals is relatively simple since the durations of the signals are not critical. The precise measurement of tone duration is, of course, critical when measuring the temporal summation process. Since these bursts must also be shaped to avoid transients, the problem of specifying the signal duration is encountered. To specify the durations of short tone bursts with altered rise- and fall-times in an unambiguous manner, Dallos and Olsen (1964) introduced the concept of *equivalent duration.* The equivalent duration of a shaped tone burst is specified by the equation:

$$t = 2r/3 + P$$

where t is the equivalent duration in milliseconds, r is the rise- and fall-times (these must be equal), and P is the stimulus peak time. The calculated equivalent duration of a shaped tone burst has the same energy content as a rectangular burst (instantaneous rise- and fall-times) of an equivalent duration. Figure 4.28 shows the stimulus envelopes for two shaped tone bursts with equivalent durations of 20 msec and a rectangular tone burst, also of 20 msec duration.

Experiment 5: Temporal Summation at the Audible Threshold

The present experiment is designed to investigate the temporal summation process for threshold level stimuli. The stimuli will be tone bursts at frequencies of 500, 1,000, 2,000, and 4,000 Hz. The equivalent durations of the bursts will be 10, 20, 40, 80, 160, 320, and 1,000 msec. All tones will have rise- and fall-times of 5 msec. The tones will be presented monaurally.

Equipment Arrangement In the present experiment thresholds will be determined using the tracking method. Therefore, the attenuator in Figure 4.29 is of the recording type. The subject is provided with a switch in the test room which controls the attenuation value at any instant in time. The

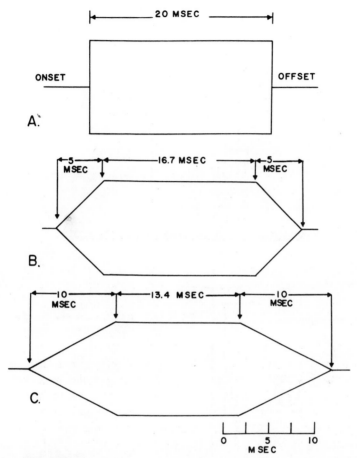

Figure 4.28. Stimulus envelopes for three tone bursts with 20 msec-equivalent durations. The upper burst (*A*) has an instantaneous rise- and fall-time. Tone bursts *B* and *C* have rise- and fall-times of 5 and 10 msec, respectively. The equivalent durations of *B* and *C* have been adjusted to the Dallos and Olsen model. From Dallos and Olsen (1964).

attenuation rate is set to 2 dB/second. It should be noted that, in this arrangement, the oscilloscope is considered to be a permanent part of the circuit. This, of course, is to monitor the shapes and durations of the tone bursts.

Calibration Calibration of the intensities in the present design is essentially unchanged from those designs previously presented. The electronic switch is placed in a "constant on" position. The oscillator is placed

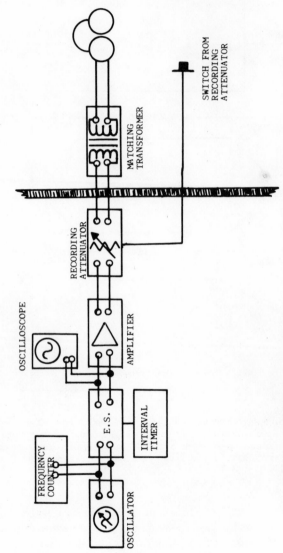

Figure 4.29. Block diagram for equipment used in Experiment 5. Temporal Integration at threshold.

at one of the four test frequencies and adjusted to produce an adequate driving voltage to the electronic switch. The electronic switch output voltage is then adjusted to yield an adequate driving voltage to the amplifier. At this point the recording attenuator is set to 0-dB attenuation and the earphone placed in the artificial ear. The gain on the amplifier is then adjusted to yield an arbitrary SPL at the test earphone. In this case the SPL is set to 70 dB for all test frequencies. The voltage producing the desired SPL is noted at either the attenuator output or across the earphone. The threshold level for any given test condition is then taken as the median value of the tracking excursions (in dB attenuation) subtracted from 70 dB SPL.

Calibration of the signal durations is accomplished using either a storage or triggered oscilloscope. As indicated, the present design calls for rise- and fall-times of 5 msec. This value is found by adjusting the appropriate rise- and fall-time control on the electronic switch so that the signal increases linearly from zero amplitude to full amplitude in 5 msec. Once this setting has been made the peak durations of the stimuli are determined. The peak times are adjusted in accordance with the Dallos and Olsen (1964) equation:

$$t = 2r/3 + P$$

Since two-thirds of r in this instance is 3.3 msec, this value must be added to the calculated peak times in order to yield the desired equivalent duration. For example, if the equivalent duration is to be set at 40 msec, the peak time of the stimulus envelope must be 36.7 msec. If the equivalent duration is to be 160 msec, the peak time would be 156.7 msec, and so on.

The interstimulus interval between tone bursts for all test conditions is to be set at 500 msec. Thus, the repetition rate of the stimuli is about 1/second.

Procedure The subject is told that he will hear short-duration tones which are pulsed on and off. He is given the attenuator switch and instructed to keep the switch pressed whenever the tone is audible and to release the switch whenever the tone is inaudible. One of the test frequencies is then set. The durations for each test frequency are to be presented in order, with the longer duration tones being presented first. Tracking for each test duration lasts for a period of 2 minutes. The next duration is then set, and tracking begins again. The experiment requires four test sessions, each corresponding to threshold determinations for the four test frequencies.

The thresholds may be plotted in a number of ways. The first is simply to plot the thresholds using the obtained SPL values. If presented in this manner, the ordinate of the temporal summation function is in dB SPL, and the abscissa is equivalent duration (plotted logarithmically). Another method is to normalize the data relative to one of the thresholds (see Figure 4.27). Either the longest or shortest tones are typically used as the reference points. This method of plotting allows for direct comparisons between the temporal summation functions for different stimulus frequencies.

Temporal Summation of Loudness

Temporal summation of loudness refers to the process by which the loudness of short-duration sounds increases as the stimulus duration increases. Two different methods have been used to investigate this relation. One approach is to have subjects perform equal loudness balances between a relatively long standard stimulus of a given SPL or SL and several shorter duration comparison stimuli (Miller, 1948; Small, Brandt, and Cox, 1962). This method permits the direct plotting of contours which relate sound pressure levels for equal loudness to stimulus duration. The other approach is to scale loudness for different duration stimuli (Ekman, Berglund, and Berglund, 1966; Stevens and Hall, 1966) using scaling procedures such as Magnitude Estimation. Contours which relate equal loudness for various duration stimuli may be obtained indirectly by noting which sound pressure levels produce equivalent scale values.

The above studies have shown that the overall form of the relation between SPL necessary for equivalent loudness and duration is the same whether obtained by loudness balancing or by scaling. In general, the SPL increases linearly as the stimulus duration is reduced below a critical duration. At stimulus durations above this critical point the loudness judgments become independent of stimulus duration. In other words, loudness increases as stimulus duration increases to a critical duration point. Above this critical point loudness is unrelated to duration.

In a study designed to investigate the relation between loudness and duration, Small, Brandt, and Cox (1962) instructed subjects to adjust the loudness of white-noise bursts of varying duration (0.5–500 msec) to the loudness of a standard 500-msec noise burst. (The spectrum of bursts of white-noise does not vary as a function of the duration of the sound. Therefore, the signals do not have to be shaped as with pure tones.) The standard noise bursts were set at either 10, 35, or 60 dB SL. A Method of Adjustment was used in which the subjects adjusted an attenuator to achieve the loudness balance. Figure 4.30 shows the results of the study.

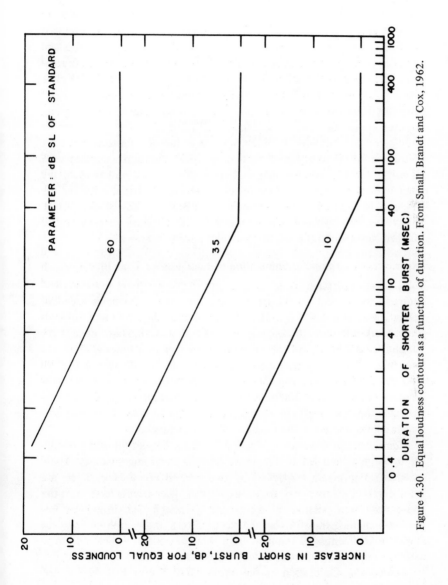

Figure 4.30. Equal loudness contours as a function of duration. From Small, Brandt and Cox, 1962.

The mean data points for each of the three standard SLs have been normalized relative to the 500-msec comparison stimulus. Two relations are evident from the figure. The first is that the trading relation between loudness and duration is unaffected by the level of the standard stimulus. Thus, the temporal summation slopes for all three standard SLs are identical. The second relation is that the value of the critical duration point decreases as the stimulus intensity increases. It is about 50 msec when the standard stimulus is at 10 dB SL and decreases to about 15 msec when the standard is set to 60 dB SL. The reader should bear in mind, however, that, although it has been generally found that the slope of the trading relation between loudness level and duration remains relatively invariant with intensity and that the critical duration increases with intensity, there is considerable scatter among various studies as to the exact numerical values of these relations. The most typical value for the temporal integration slope is roughly 10 dB/decade (Zwislocki, 1969). This value, of course, would represent a direct inverse proportionality between stimulus duration decreases and intensity increases.

Experiment 6:   Temporal Summation of Loudness for Tone Bursts

The present experiment is designed to investigate temporal summation of loudness for several sound frequencies. The test frequencies are 500, 1,000, 2,000, and 4,000 Hz. The experimental method is to have subjects perform equal loudness balances between a 500-msec standard tone (at 20, 50, and 80 dB SPL) and several comparison duration tones at the same frequency. The comparison durations will be 10, 20, 50, 100, 200, 500, 1,000, and 2,000 msec. The tone pairs will be heard monaurally and will be separated in time by 500 msec. An interstimulus interval of 2.5 seconds separates the tone pairs. In all instances the loudness of the comparison tone is adjusted to equal the loudness of the standard tone.

Equipment Arrangement   Figure 4.31 shows the output of the oscillator to be split and led to the inputs of two electronic switches. These switches, in turn, are controlled by two interval timers. The timers are wired together so that they trigger each other. The outputs from both the upper and lower portions of the circuit are mixed, fed through an impedance-matching transformer, and then led to a single earphone. Attenuator 1 (experimenter's attenuator) is within the control room, and attenuator 2 (subject's attenuator) is in the subject's test chamber.

Calibration   Calibration of the output SPLs is essentially unchanged from those designs in which the outputs from two channels have been mixed. In the present design the standard tone SPLs will be 20, 50, and 80 dB. Therefore, it is advisable that the output SPL of the upper channel

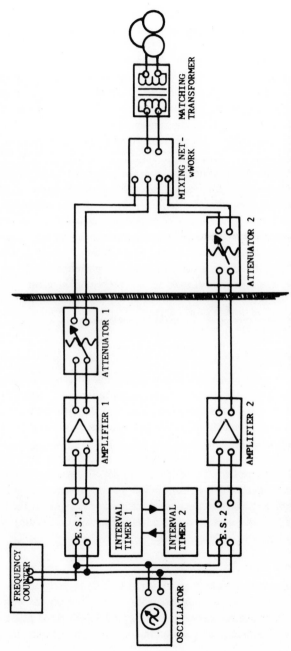

Figure 4.31. Block diagram for the equipment used in Experiment 6. Temporal Summation of Loudness.

(standard channel) be set to 100 dB SPL with no attenuation present using attenuator 1. Attenuation values of 80, 50, and 20 dB will then produce the 20, 50, and 80 dB SPL tones, respectively. Calibration of the lower (comparison) channel is identical to that of the upper channel. The attenuation value at which the loudness balance is made is then simply subtracted from 100 dB SPL in order to obtain the comparison tone SPL.

Signal durations will be adjusted using the Dallos and Olsen (1964) equation. Rise- and fall-times of the tones will be 5 msec.

Procedure The subject is instructed that he will hear pairs of tones which are separated by a short time interval. Furthermore, he is told that he cannot change the loudness of the first tone, but can change the loudness of the second tone using his attenuator. In order to make a loudness match the subject is free to hear as many pairs of tones as he feels is necessary. When a match is made the subject signals the experimenter. The experimenter then reads the subject's attenuator setting (either visually through the observation window or electrically using a voltmeter wired across the subject's earphone terminals). Eight comparison durations for the three standard intensity levels are presented in a random order during a test session for one test frequency. Four sessions, one for each test frequency, are included in the design.

4.5. MASKING

Masking refers to the process by which the audible threshold of one sound (signal) is raised by the simultaneous presentation of a second sound (masker). The degree of masking is expressed as the difference in decibels between the signal threshold in silence and that obtained when the masker is present. Thus, for example, a 35-dB *threshold shift* refers to the difference in threshold in quiet versus the threshold in the presence of a masker which increases the threshold by 35 dB. The *masked threshold* is the level of the signal which is just audible in the presence of the masker. Just about any type of sound may serve either as the signal or the masker. However, much of the work in the area has been concerned with pure tone masking by either noise or other tones.

Masking of Pure Tones by White-Noise

In their classic paper, Hawkins and Stevens (1950) investigated the masking effects of white-noise on pure tone thresholds. Thresholds were determined for 16 frequencies between 100 Hz and 9,000 Hz in quiet and at eight noise levels. Subjects were seated in a quiet room and were instructed to adjust a variable attenuator so that the tones were just audible. All measurements were monaural.

Figure 4.32 shows the results obtained by Hawkins and Stevens (1950) in the form of masked threshold contours. Each contour shows the monaural thresholds for the pure tones (in dB SPL) when masked by white-noise at a given intensity level. The parameter of the figure is spectrum level. The reader will recall that the spectrum level of any noise which is flat and continuous is defined as the SPL present within a one cycle (1 Hz) bandwidth of the noise. Spectrum level may be calculated using the equation:

$$\text{dB SPL/Hz (spectrum level)} = \text{overall SPL} - 10 \log_{10} \text{BW}$$

where BW is the bandwidth of the noise. Hawkins and Stevens (1950) did not report the overall SPLs of their masking noises. However, they did report the noise bandwidth to be about 9,000 Hz. The value $10 \log_{10}$ 9,000 is nearly 40 dB. Therefore, the overall noise SPLs can be estimated as ranging from 30–100 dB in 10-dB increments. Several relations are seen in the figure. The first is that at low noise levels the thresholds of tones located in the midfrequency range (about 1,000–4,000 Hz) are shifted by a greater amount than those frequencies above and below this region. Thus, the masked threshold contours at these low masking levels appear to be influenced by the threshold curve in silence. A second feature is that, as the masking level increases, the contours become flatter. This, of course, indicates that the SPLs necessary to reach the masked threshold are independent of stimulus frequency at high masking levels. Finally, it is seen for all masked frequencies, except in the region of the threshold in silence, that an increase in the masking noise will produce an equivalent threshold shift.

The masked threshold contours seen in Figure 4.32 supported the notion of a *critical band* as presented by Fletcher and Munson (1933) and Fletcher (1940). The critical band concept was based upon two assumptions. The first was that a tone masked by noise was masked only by a narrow "critical band" of frequencies whose center corresponded to the tone being masked. Frequency components of the noise lying outside the critical band contributed little or nothing to the masking. The second assumption was that, when a tone was just audible above the noise, the total energy within the critical band was equivalent to the energy of the tone.

Hawkins and Stevens (1950) were able to estimate the critical bandwidths at various frequencies by noting the ratio (in dB) between the

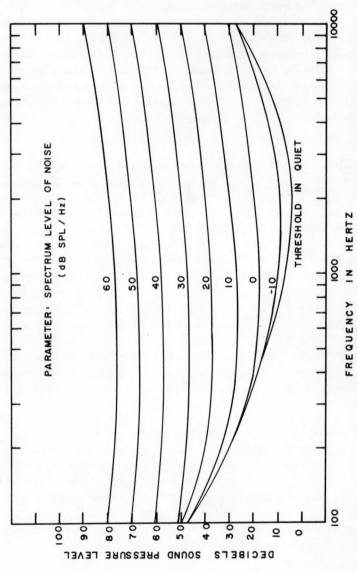

Figure 4.32. Masked-threshold contours for pure tones in white-noise. The parameter of the figure is the spectrum level of the noise. From Hawkins and Stevens (1950).

masked threshold SPLs and the spectrum level of the noise. Since both units are logarithmic the ratio could simply be calculated by subtracting the dB SPL/Hz of the noise from the dB SPL value associated with the masked threshold of the tone. These values were averaged over the four top contours in Figure 4.32 for each of the 16 test frequencies.

Figure 4.33 shows the width of the critical band both in dB (left-hand ordinate) and in Hz (right-hand ordinate) as a function of frequency. The dB values were calculated in the manner specified above. The bandwidths in Hz were calculated by assuming an equivalency between the energy levels present in the critical band and the masked tone. For example, at 1,000 Hz the masked threshold is 18 dB greater than the spectrum level of the noise. An 18-dB energy difference corresponds to a 63:1 ratio. Therefore the bandwidth of the critical band is calculated to be 63 Hz wide. To further illustrate, note that the width of the critical band at 10,000 Hz is 28 dB. As 28 dB corresponds to an energy ratio of 630:1, it may be assumed that the critical bandwidth at this frequency is 630 Hz wide, or extending from 9,685 Hz to 10,315 Hz. The critical band, as calculated in this indirect manner, has in recent years been more appropriately termed the *critical ratio*. Scharf (1970) notes that the calculated critical ratios are about 2.5 times smaller than determinations of critical bands made using more direct approaches, such as when the bandwidths of narrow noise bands are systematically increased. The critical ratio values do, however, parallel the critical band values as a function of frequency.

Figure 4.34 shows the relation between masking (M) and the *effective level* of the masking noise (Z). The plotted function represents the best-fit solution for six test frequencies (350, 500, 1,000, 2,800, 4,000, and 5,600 Hz). M is the difference between the threshold level obtained under quiet conditions and that obtained under the various noise levels. Z is the difference in dB between the pure tone threshold in quiet and the total energy in the critical band at the masked threshold level. Since the energy present in the critical band is assumed to equal that of the masked pure tone, Z may be considered to be the sensation level of the critical band. Note that at effective levels above 0 dB the slope of the function is unity. Thus, a constant signal-to-noise ratio is maintained at the masked threshold for each of the test frequencies.

Masking of Pure Tones by Pure Tones

The masking of one pure tone upon another may be considered to be the antithesis of white-noise masking. White-noise is continuous and flat in its spectrum. A pure tone has a line spectrum in that its entire energy is concentrated at only one frequency. Therefore, it is to be expected that

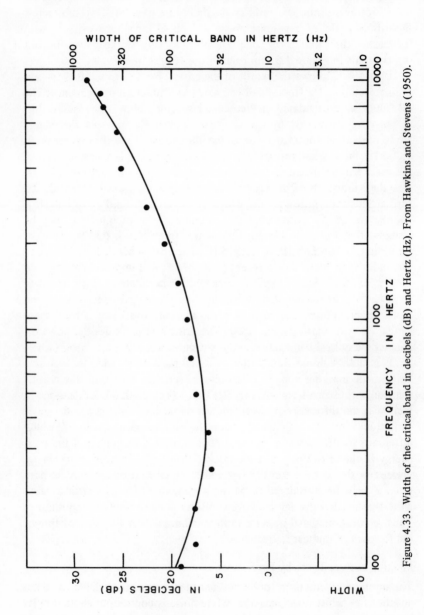

Figure 4.33. Width of the critical band in decibels (dB) and Hertz (Hz). From Hawkins and Stevens (1950).

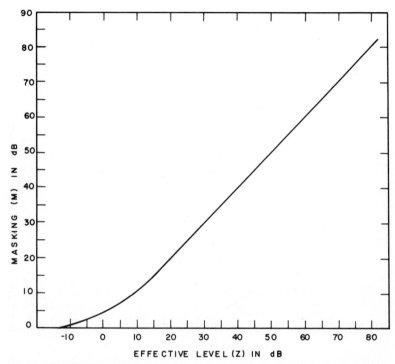

Figure 4.34. Relation between masking (*M*) and effective level (*Z*) of the masking noise. From Hawkins and Stevens, 1950.

fundamental differences will exist between masking patterns produced by the two masker types.

Wegel and Lane (1924) were the first to use electronic instrumentation to obtain pure tone masking patterns. The maskers were pure tones set to either 200, 400, 800, 1,200, 2,400, or 3,600 Hz. Sensation levels of the maskers varied between 20 and 100 dB in 20-dB steps.

Figure 4.35 shows the masking patterns obtained by Wegel and Lane (1924) using a 1,200-Hz masker at five sensation levels. The ordinate of the figure is the amount of threshold shift (in dB) found at the various test frequencies. Several relations are seen in the figure. First, at the lowest sensation levels (20 and 40 dB), the shapes of the masking patterns are symmetrical about the masker frequency. However, as the intensity of the masker increases above 60-dB SL, the masking patterns become asymmetrical, with the masking effect increasing rapidly toward the higher frequencies. Another feature of the figure is the dips in the patterns at the masker frequency (1,200 Hz) and at integral multiples of that frequency.

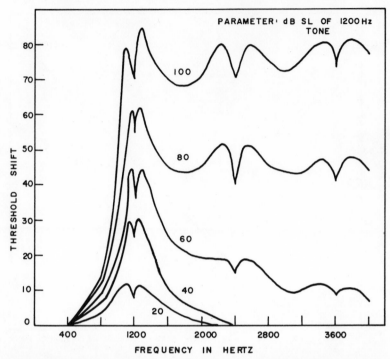

Figure 4.35. Masking pattern of a 1,200-pure tone masker on the threshold of other sound frequencies. The parameter of the figure is the sensation level of the masker. From Wegel and Lane (1924).

These dips become more pronounced as the sensation level of the masker increases. The dips have been attributed to beating between harmonics of the masker frequency and other test frequencies caused by nonlinear distortion in the cochlea. Notice also that, at the higher sensation levels, depressions or "troughs" are present between the masker frequency and its harmonics.

Ehmer (1959a) extended the work of the earlier investigators. Subjects were presented with pure tone maskers between 250 Hz and 8,000 Hz (in octave steps). The sensation levels of the maskers varied from 20–100 dB. Subjects tracked their thresholds using a Bekesy audiometer which swept frequency at a rate of either one octave in 2 or 4 minutes. The signals were pulsed on and off for a period of 200 msec each. The masking tones were on continuously and were electronically mixed with the pulsed tones. All listening was monaural.

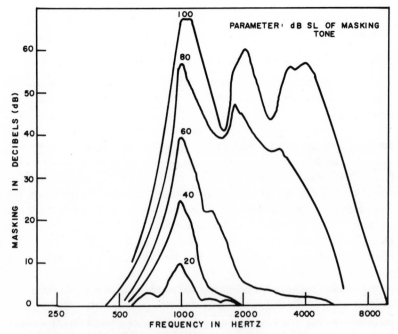

Figure 4.36. Masking of pure tones by a 1,000-Hz tone. The parameter is the sensation level of the 1,000-Hz masker. From Ehmer (1959*a*).

Figure 4.36 shows the results obtained by Ehmer (1959*a*) using a 1,000-Hz masker. The ordinate of the figure is, once again, masking in dB. The abscissa shows the frequencies of the masked tones. Sensation levels of the masker are indicated on the individual functions. Ehmer's results are similar to those obtained by Wegel and Lane (1924) in that at the two lowest sensation levels the masking functions are symmetrical about the masker. At sensation levels of 60 dB and above, the patterns become asymmetrical because of the failure of the masking to spread to frequencies below the masker. Ehmer's results differ from those in the earlier study in that the dips in the masking patterns are not found at harmonics of the masker. Furthermore, peaks in the patterns are seen which migrate toward the second and third harmonics of the masker as the sensation level is increased. Only when the masker level reaches 100 dB SL does the second peak correspond with the second harmonic (2,000 Hz) of the masker. Ehmer indicated that the masking pattern elicited by a pure tone stimulus probably results from the activity pattern set up along the basilar membrane. Cochlear patterns elicited by tones have been shown to be asymmetrical in much the same fashion as the tone on tone masking patterns.

Masking of Pure Tones by Narrow Bands of Noise

Tone on tone masking patterns are subject to the influence of audible beats and difference tones caused by the interaction of the pure tone stimuli. Ehmer (1959*a*) reported that, when a pure tone masker is used, the masked tones maintain their tonal quality at all frequencies except in the region of the masker and its harmonics. In the region of the masker two types of beats are perceived. At signal frequencies close to the masker (or its harmonics), wavering beats are heard, the rate of which is determined by the frequency difference between the tones. As the frequency separation increases between the masker and the masked tone, fused beats are heard which give the sound a rough quality. To avoid these influences, several investigators (Carter and Kryter, 1962; Egan and Hake, 1950; Ehmer, 1959*b*) have replaced the pure tone masker with a narrow band of noise.

Egan and Hake (1950) compared the masking patterns produced by a band of noise 90 Hz wide and centered at 410 Hz with a 400-Hz pure tone masker. The test frequencies vaired between 100 Hz and 6,000 Hz. The levels of the maskers varied from 40–80 dB SPL in 20-dB steps. The results of their study showed the masking patterns to be smoother for the noise bands than for the pure tone maskers. That is, the noise bands did not reflect the influence of audible beats and difference tones. Second, when the two masker types were set at the same overall SPL of 80 dB (see Egan and Hake, 1950, Figure 7), the noise band produced considerably more masking within the band than did the tone at closely adjacent frequencies. The amount of extended masking, however, was similar to that produced by the pure tone masker.

Ehmer (1959*b*) extended the work of the earlier investigators. In this study masking patterns were obtained for pure tone maskers at 500, 1,000, 2,000, and 4,000 Hz (at 60 and 80 dB SL) and for noise bands of equal intensity and centered at the same four frequencies. The noise bands were $\frac{1}{3}$-octave wide. Subjects tracked their thresholds using a Bekesy audiometer. The maskers were constantly on and were electronically mixed with the pulsed (200 msec on and off) tones. All listening was monaural.

Figure 4.37 shows the masking patterns obtained when both the tone and the center frequency of the noise band were set to 1,000 Hz and had an overall SPL of 87 dB. Also shown in the figure are the subjects' absolute thresholds in quiet (lowermost curve) and the frequency response

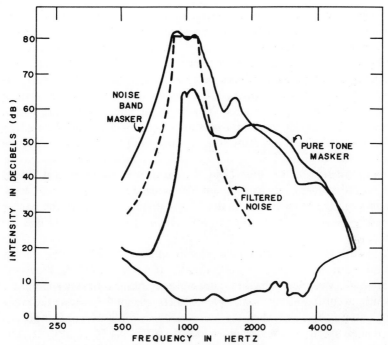

Figure 4.37. Masked thresholds for tones versus noise bands. From Ehmer (1959b).

of the band-pass filter. Note that the frequency limits of the noise are 880 and 1,150 Hz, and that the spectrum level of the noise is nearly 63 dB (dB SPL/Hz = 87 − 10 log$_{10}$ 270 = 62.7). The figure shows clearly that, within the pass-band of the noise, there is considerably more masking than produced by the pure tone masker. This presumably is because the noise does not interact with the masked tones as in the case of pure tone maskers. Notice also that the masking pattern for noise meets the pure tone masking pattern at the second peak of the latter. Thereafter, the masking effect for the two maskers types approximate one another.

It will be recalled from the work of Wegel and Lane (1924) and Ehmer (1959a) that a pure tone masker is highly effective at masking frequencies higher than itself. On the other hand, the masking effect at frequencies lower than the masker is minimal. This is not the case for narrow noise bands when the masking level is set to relatively high intensity levels (Bilger and Hirsh, 1956; Spieth, 1957).

Bilger and Hirsh (1956) were the first to identify what they termed *"remote masking."* In their study, 11 bands of noise, each corresponding to a pitch interval of 250 mels, were used as the maskers. The overall SPLs of the noise bands were set at either 40, 60, 80, or 100 dB. The slopes of the noise bands were adjusted to fall off at a rate of either 36 or 54 dB/octave. Subjects tracked their thresholds using a modified Bekesy technique. The pure tone signals were switched on and off three times/second without audible transients. The results indicated that the masked thresholds closely approximated the slope of the filtered noise for frequencies at the center of the noise bands and downward whenever the masking noise was relatively low. However, as the overall level of the noise band was raised to 80 or 100 dB SPL, a spread of masking occurred on the downward side of the noise band. This remote masking did not fall off toward the lower frequencies, but rather remained at a constant level, paralleling the audiogram in quiet. Furthermore, the amount of remote masking was not found to be linearly related to the level of the masking noise.

Spieth (1957) confirmed the presence of remote masking using narrow bands of noise centered at 500, 1,000, 2,000, and 4,000 Hz. Pure tone thresholds were determined in quiet and noise using a Bekesy audiometer which swept frequency from 100–9,000 Hz. Figure 4.38 shows the masking patterns obtained when the noise band was centered at 1,000 Hz and the noise spectrum levels were set to either 40, 60, or 76 dB SPL/Hz. Also shown in the figure are the average pure tone thresholds in quiet (*bottom curve*) and the spectrum of the noise at maximum intensity (*dashed line function*). The figure clearly shows the presence of remote masking for all three noise levels.

Deatherage, Davis, and Eldridge (1957) demonstrated a physiological basis for remote masking. Observations were made on guinea pigs with intracochlear electrodes. They showed that either an amplitude-modulated (AM) high frequency tone (6,950 Hz) or a high frequency pass-band of noise centered at 6,950 Hz, when raised to a sufficiently high level, produced a cochlear microphonic (CM) in the apical (low frequency) region of the cochlea in addition to the expected CM in the basal region. They attributed this to a nonlinearity of the ear at high intensity levels. The ear detects the envelope of the masker whether it is random (as in the case of the noise) or periodic (as in the case of the AM-modulated tone). It is this low frequency detection which is effective in the masking of low frequency sounds by higher frequency maskers.

Experiment 7: Masking of Pure Tones by White-Noise

Equipment Arrangement The equipment arrangement shown in Figure 4.39 consists of two separate branches whose outputs are mixed just

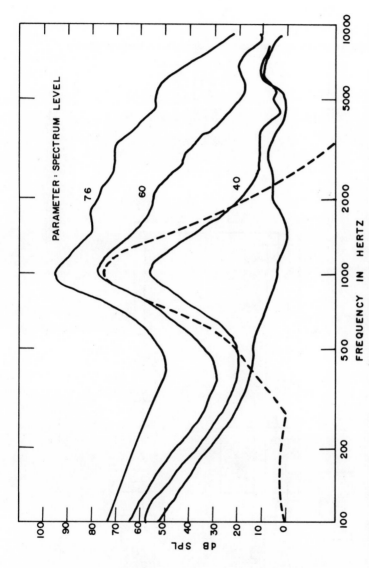

Figure 4.38. Masking patterns for a band of noise centered at 1,000 Hz. The parameter of the figure is the spectrum level of the noise. Also shown are the pure tone thresholds in quiet (*bottom curve*) and spectrum of the noise at the highest noise level. From Spieth (1957).

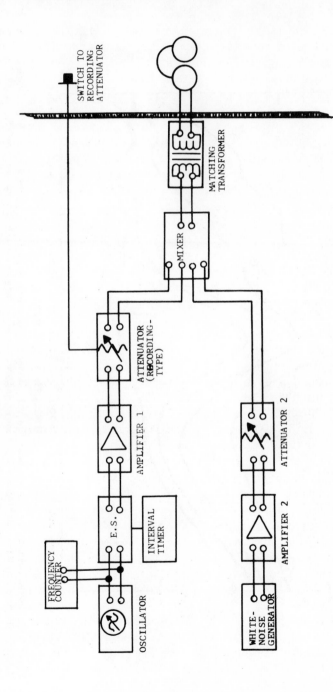

Figure 4.39. Block diagram for the equipment used in Experiment 7.

before the earphone. The upper portion of the circuit generates the pure tone stimuli while the lower portion generates the white-noise. Specifically, the output of the oscillator is fed to the input of the electronic switch. The switch is placed in a mode where it automatically turns the tone on and off. It is decided that the on- and off-times will be 500 msec each. The rise- and fall-times of the tone bursts will be 25 msec. The output from the switch is then passed through an amplifier, a recording attenuator, and then to the mixer. The noise circuit consists of a white-noise generator, an amplifier, and an attenuator. The attenuator output is mixed with the pulsed tones and delivered to the earphone. The test frequencies will be 125, 250, 500, 750, 1,000, 1,500, 2,000, 3,000, 4,000, 6,000 and 8,000 Hz. The overall SPLs of the noise will be 30, 60, and 90 dB.

Calibration The tone circuit may be calibrated in much the same manner as previous designs. It is recommended that a 1,000-Hz tone be first set to 100 dB SPL. The other test frequencies are then calibrated by noting the SPLs produced at the earphone when the oscillator frequency is changed. Since a typical earphone used in the laboratory is not flat in its response over the entire auditory range, it is to be expected that the output SPLs will change. These values are noted and used for determinations of the threshold levels. For example, if, at 6,000 Hz, the SPL produced at the earphone is 96 dB, this value minus the attenuator setting on attenuator 1 is the obtained threshold level. It must be remembered, however, that the voltage at 1,000 Hz (V_3, V_4, or V_5) must always produce 100 dB SPL in order for the other frequencies to remain in calibration. If this dB value varies in any direction, the other frequencies will change an equivalent amount.

The noise circuit may be calibrated by raising the noise generator voltage (V_6) to adequately drive amplifier 2. Attenuator 2 is then set to 0-dB attenuation and attenuator 1 set to maximum attenuation. The amplifier gain is then adjusted so that the desired SPL is produced at the earphone. In this instance the level is adjusted to 90 dB SPL. The voltage producing this output is noted at either V_5, V_7, or V_8. The other noise levels may be obtained by introducing an appropriate attenuation value.

Procedure The subject is seated in a quiet room and is given the switch to the recording attenuator. The subject is instructed to press the switch whenever a pulsing tone is present and to release the switch when the tone is inaudible. The experiment consists of four test sessions. In three of the test sessions thresholds are determined for all 11 test frequencies under one of the three noise conditions. In the fourth session the tones are tracked in quiet (attenuator 2 set to maximum attenuation). The noise level to be used and the presentation sequence of the test frequencies are randomly determined. Subjects track their thresholds for 1.5 minutes at each frequency. The attenuation rate is set at 2 dB/second.

The results of the study may be plotted in a number of ways. However, for direct comparison with the Hawkins and Stevens (1950) masking function (Figure 4.32), the ordinate should be the frequency of the masked tones. Spectrum levels of the white-noise may be calculated in the manner described earlier.

REFERENCES

American National Standards Institute (ANSI). 1969. Specifications for Audiometers. S3.6.

Bilger, R. C., and I. J. Hirsh. 1956. Masking of tones by bands of noise. J. Acoust. Soc. Amer. 28: 623–630.

Carter, N. L., and K. D. Kryter. 1962. Masking of pure tones and speech. J. Aud. Res. 2: 66–98.

Churcher, B. G. 1935. A loudness scale for industrial noise measurements. J. Acoust. Soc. Amer. 6: 216–226.

Cohen, A. 1961. Further investigation of the effects of intensity upon the pitch of pure tones. J. Acoust. Soc. Amer. 33: 1,363–1,376.

Corso, J. F. 1965. Air conduction thresholds for high frequency tones. Paper presented at the Eastern Psychological Association, Atlantic City, N. J.

Dallos, P. J., and W. O. Olsen. 1964. Integration of energy at threshold with gradual rise-fall pips. J. Acoust. Soc. Amer. 36: 743–751.

Deatherage, B. H., H. Davis, and D. H. Eldridge. 1957. Physiological evidence for the masking of low frequencies by high. J. Acoust. Soc. Amer. 29: 132–137.

Doughty, J. M., and W. R. Garner. 1947. Pitch characteristics of short tones. I. Two kinds of pitch thresholds. J. Exp. Psychol. 37: 351–365.

Egan, J. P. and H. W. Hake. 1950. On the masking pattern of a simple auditory stimulus. J. Acoust. Soc. Amer. 22: 622–630.

Ehmer, R. H. 1959a. Masking patterns of tones. J. Acoust. Soc. Amer. 31: 1,115–1,120.

Ehmer, R. H. 1959b. Masking by tones vs noise bands. J. Acoust. Soc. Amer. 31: 1,153–1,156.

Ekman, E., G. Berglund, and V. Berglund. 1966. Loudness as a function of duration of auditory stimulation. Scand. J. Psychol. 7: 201–208.

Fletcher, H. 1940. Auditory patterns. Rev. Modern Physics 12: 47–65.

Fletcher, H., and W. A. Munson. 1933. Loudness, its definition, measurement, and calibration. J. Acoust. Soc. Amer. 5: 82–108.

Garner, W. R. 1947. The effect of frequency spectrum on temporal integration of energy in the ear. J. Acoust. Soc. Amer. 19: 808–815.

Garner, W. R., and G. A. Miller. 1947. The masked threshold of pure tones as a function of duration. J. Exp. Psychol. 37: 293–303.

Harris, J. D. 1952. Pitch discrimination. J. Acoust. Soc. Amer. 24: 750–755.

Harris, J. D., and C. K. Myers. 1971. Tentative audiometric threshold-level standards from 8 through 18 kiloHertz. J. Acoust. Soc. Amer. 49: 600–601.

Hawkins, J. E., Jr., and S. S. Stevens. 1950. The masking of pure tones and of speech by white noise. J. Acoust. Soc. Amer. 22: 6–13.

Hellman, R. P., and J. J. Zwislocki. 1963. Monaural loudness function of a 1,000-cps tone and interaural summation. J. Acoust. Soc. Amer. 35: 856–865.

International Organization for Standardization (ISO). 1959. Expression of the Physical and Subjective Magnitudes of Sound or Noise. ISO/ R131–1959.

International Organization for Standardization (ISO). 1964. Reference Zero for Pure Tone Audiometers. ISO/ R389–1964.

Licklider, J. C. R. 1951. Basic Correlates of the Auditory Stimulus. In S. S. Stevens (ed.), Handbook of Experimental Psychology, pp. 985–1,039. John Wiley & Sons, Inc., New York.

Miller, G. A. 1948. The perception of short bursts of noise. J. Acoust. Soc. Amer. 20: 160–170.

Morgan, C. T., W. R. Garner, and R. Galambos. 1951. Pitch and intensity. J. Acoust. Soc. Amer. 23: 658–663.

Olsen, W. O., and R. Carhart. 1966. Integration of acoustic power at threshold by normal listeners. J. Acoust. Soc. Amer. 40: 591–599.

Peterson, A. P. G., and E. E. Gross. 1972. Handbook of Noise Measurement, pp. 248–249. General Radio, Concord, Mass.

Reisz, R. R. 1928. Differential intensity sensitivity of the ear for pure tones. Physics Rev. 31: 867–875.

Robinson, D. W., and R. S. Dadson. 1956. A re-determination of equal-loudness relations for pure tones. Brit. J. Applied Physics 7: 166–181.

Scharf, B. 1970. Critical Bands. In J. V. Tobias (ed.), Foundations of Modern Auditory Theory, Volume 1, pp. 157–202. Academic Press, Inc., New York.

Shower, E. G., and R. Biddulph. 1931. Differential pitch sensitivity of the ear. J. Acoust. Soc. Amer. 3: 275–287.

Small, A. M., Jr., J. F. Brandt, and P. G. Cox. 1962. Loudness as a function of signal duration. J. Acoust. Soc. Amer. 34: 513–514.

Spieth, W. 1957. Downward spread of masking. J. Acoust. Soc. Amer. 29: 502–505.

Stevens, J. C., and J. W. Hall. 1966. Brightness and loudness as functions of stimulus duration. Percept. & Psychophysics. 1: 319–327.

Stevens, S. S. 1935. The relation of pitch to intensity. J. Acoust. Soc. Amer. 6: 150–154.

Stevens, S. S. 1936. A scale for the measurement of a psychological magnitude: Loudness. Psychol. Rev. 43: 405–416.

Stevens, S. S. 1951. Mathematics, Measurement, and Psychophysics. In S. S. Stevens (ed.), Handbook of Experimental Psychology, pp. 1–49. John Wiley & Sons, New York.

Stevens, S. S. 1956. The direct estimation of sensory magnitudes—loudness. Amer. J. Psychol. 69: 1—25.

Stevens, S. S. 1957a. Concerning the form of the loudness function. J. Acoust. Soc. Amer. 29: 603—606.

Stevens, S. S. 1957b. On the psychophysical law. Psychol. Rev. 64: 153—181.

Stevens, S. S. 1958. Problems and methods of psychophysics. Psychol. Bull. 54: 177—196.

Stevens, S. S., J. Volkmann, and E. B. Newman. 1937. A scale for the measurement of the psychological magnitude pitch. J. Acoust. Soc. Amer. 8: 185—190.

Stevens, S. S., and J. Volkmann. 1940. The relation of pitch to frequency: A revised scale. Amer. J. Psychol. 53: 329—353.

Wegel, R. L., and C. E. Lane. 1924. The auditory masking of one pure tone by another and its probable relation to the dynamics of the inner ear. Physics Rev. 23: 266—285.

Zwislocki, J. J. 1969. Temporal summation of loudness: An anylysis. J. Acoust. Soc. Amer. 46: 431—441.

index